Plastic Surgery

PLASTIC SURGERY

~

*What You Need to Know—Before,
During, and After*

Richard A. Marfuggi, M.D., F.A.C.S.

A Perigee Book

A Perigee Book
Published by The Berkley Publishing Group
A division of Penguin Putnam Inc.
375 Hudson Street
New York, NY 10014

Copyright © 1998 by Dr. Richard A. Marfuggi
Book design by Jenny Drossin
Cover design by Dorothy Wachtenheim
Interior photographs by Richard A. Marfuggi, M.D., and Michael E. Valdes, M.D.
Interior illustrations by James A. Zulauf

First edition: February 1998

Published simultaneously in Canada.

The Penguin Putnam Inc. World Wide Web site address is
http://www.penguinputnam.com

Library of Congress Cataloging-in-Publication Data

Marfuggi, Richard A.
Plastic surgery : what you need to know—before, during,
and after / Richard A. Marfuggi.
p.   cm.
"A Perigee book."
Includes bibliographical references.
ISBN 0-399-52374-X
1. Surgery, Plastic—Popular works. I. Title.
RD118.M376   1998
617.9′5—dc21   97-15709
                                                                    CIP

Printed in the United States of America

10 9 8 7 6 5 4 3

For Andrew

Contents

~

PART ONE

Your Introduction to Plastic Surgery

What You Must Know

PART TWO

Your Guide to Plastic Surgery Procedures

What You Should Know

Preface

~

Whenever I attend a party and word circulates that I'm a plastic surgeon, the fun begins. I've heard it all, from proclamations such as, "I would *never* have plastic surgery," or catty remarks about celebrities to blatant requests for on-the-spot consultations.

Interestingly, the concerns and questions vary little from party to party, male to female, young to old, or region to region. More than once, I wished that I had had a book to hand to these people so I wouldn't have to keep defending the specialty, dispelling rumors and myths, and attempting to give accurate, detailed, yet understandable information.

Well, finally, here it is, and you may understand why I was tempted to use the subtitle: *The Longest Cocktail Party in the World*.

In my experience, the individuals—usually women—who proclaim that they would *never* have plastic surgery hope to be convinced otherwise. They're really looking for validation or encouragement. The people who criticize a celebrity's appearance are often concerned that they would be similarly criticized if they were to have plastic surgery. Those seeking on-the-spot consultation clearly lack an understanding of the complexities of their request.

Some people try to put me on the defensive by reciting a litany of plastic surgery disasters. My standard response is, "Every horror story you've ever heard is true . . . and you probably haven't heard them all!"

I will never say that you can't have problems with a plastic surgery operation, but I assure you that there's a lot that you can do to avoid getting into trouble.

First and foremost, you must educate yourself. You—as well as your doctor—are responsible for your welfare. The era of the passive patient is over. You need to know what you are undertaking and prepare accordingly. It is my hope that this book will help you with this process, even if you ultimately decide that plastic surgery is not for you. Yes, *not* for you. Plastic surgery is not the solution for everyone. It has, however, improved the lives of many.

This book is my gift to you with the hope of giving you everything you need to know—before, during, and after plastic surgery.

Acknowledgments

~

Special thanks to my patients, who inspired this book; Sallie Batson, who helped me to write it; Pat McGraw, my office manager, who kept everything on track while we were writing it; Mitch Douglas, my diligent agent; John Duff, my dedicated editor, who made certain that our manuscript became a book; and Curt Styer and his staff at Digital Exchange, Inc., who processed our photos to mask the identities of patients.

How to Use This Book

~

This book is an offering to *all* potential plastic surgery patients. It is a guidebook that makes plastic surgery procedures understandable without minimizing the risks or maximizing the benefits.

Before you jump ahead in search of details on tummy tucks or face-lifts, let me tell you how to use this book:

Part 1: Your Introduction to Plastic Surgery

This entire section is *required* reading. It doesn't matter if you are considering laser resurfacing to improve aging skin or liposuction to rid yourself of a double chin. You *must* read this introductory section in its entirety. Like grammar school before high school, high school before college, this section provides the fundamental information you will need to make informed choices.

Armed with this basic knowledge, you are then prepared to move on to Part 2.

Part 2: Your Guide to Plastic Surgery Procedures

This section defines specific procedures in detail. *Now* you may read about those procedures you've been considering. You don't have to read every chapter, although you might want to, just for your own interest. For the most part, the chapters are organized in the following format:

Overview

A description of each operation gives you a better understanding of what can and cannot be achieved.

Definitions

To make certain you understand what you are reading, this section includes a glossary of terms specific to each procedure. There is a complete glossary of these terms at the conclusion of the book on page 227.

The Procedure

This section explains how the operation is performed, i.e., what the doctor will be doing and where incisions will be made.

Length of Procedure

This entry gives you the general times that it will take to perform each specific procedure.

Anesthesia

A full range of options, from local to general anesthesia, will be outlined.

In/Outpatient

In most cases, plastic surgery can be performed safely in a walk-in surgical facility. However, some procedures are best done in a hospital. The full range of options will be discussed.

Incisions/Scarring

If you have an incision, you *will* have a scar. It does not have to be obvious. This section discusses incision placement as well as wound care, a subject vital to keeping obvious scarring to the minimum.

Pain

This section will describe how much pain and discomfort you can realistically expect after your operation, and how it will be managed.

Specific Risks

There is always an element of risk in any operation. Although basic risks are explained in this introductory section (see page 7), we will also discuss the risks specific for each procedure.

Recovery Time

This section includes a *realistic* schedule for returning to work, as well as any restrictions on exercise, sex, sun exposure, and travel.

Frequency/Duration of Results

Many procedures will last a lifetime. Others may need to be repeated or will have relatively short-term benefits. In this section, the varying degrees of permanence are reviewed.

What to Expect

This section will provide specific guidelines as to what you might expect in terms of recovery time, follow-up procedures, or care that are not specifically reviewed in other sections.

Fee Range/Insurance Coverage

In this section, I'll tell you approximately how much your procedure will cost and discuss the possibility of insurance coverage.

Important Questions to Ask

This introduction outlines *essential* questions that must be answered before you decide to have *any* plastic surgery procedure. Here, you will be given questions that relate to the specific procedure. Make certain that they are answered to *your* satisfaction.

Remember, the basics explained in Part 1 remain the same. It doesn't matter where you live or what procedure you are considering. Surgeon to surgeon, details may vary, but basics remain the same. If you consult with two surgeons about the same problem, you may get two different approaches, both equally valid. Don't confuse variations in technique with good or bad care. Plastic surgery marries medical science with art. The science is the constant; the artistic aspects account for any variation.

Your Introduction to Plastic Surgery

~

What You **Must** Know

What Is Plastic Surgery?

Perhaps the casual use of the words *plastic* and *cosmetic* have trivialized this constantly changing, rapidly evolving branch of medicine. Reconstructive surgery remains worthy, while plastic or cosmetic surgery are thought of as superficial.

In truth, both terms have most noble origins: Plastic comes from the Greek word *plastikos,* to mold or shape, while cosmetic is from *kosmos,* also Greek, meaning to order or adorn.

Early plastic surgeons treated injuries of war. The specialty expanded, applying the knowledge gained on the battlefield to include treatment of congenital defects, burns, the ravages of disease, and, finally, even the marks of time. The specialty now includes two components:

❖ *Reconstructive Plastic Surgery:* Surgical procedures that restore function are known as reconstructive plastic surgery. The goal of such operations is to repair abnormal structures of the body, be they caused by congenital defects, developmental abnormalities, trauma, infection, tumors, or disease. Reconstructive surgery is also performed to approximate normal appearance.

❖ *Cosmetic or Aesthetic Plastic Surgery:* Procedures to reshape or improve normal body structures are known as cosmetic or aesthetic plastic surgery. The goal of these operations is to enhance the patient's appearance.

Both reconstructive and cosmetic plastic surgeons strive to enhance the quality of life of their patients.

Is Plastic Surgery for You?

I suggest that just about everyone on this planet looks into the mirror and sees *one* thing that they would change about themselves if they could. They see it so clearly that, for some, it becomes the *only* thing they see. This flaw may be as subtle as a mole on the arm or as obvious as a scar on the face. The spectrum of concern for such conditions ranges from simple awareness to debilitating obsession. Such concern may lead one to the plastic surgeon.

If you see yourself in this scenario, you must first decide if this is the best course to take. Almost any physical problem that affects appearance *can* be improved with plastic surgery, but just because something is able to be done does not mean that it *should* be done.

Your first step is to examine your motives for seeking improvement of a defect, whether it is very obvious to everyone or whether it bothers only you.

Next, study your expectations, not just of how you hope you will look but also of how you expect your life to be changed once the defect is corrected.

If you want to get rid of a hump in your nose in hopes of straightening your profile, that's fine. If you hope to get rid of a hump in your nose to get a date, plastic surgery is not the answer.

If you want to have your breasts enlarged in order to feel more comfortable about your body, that's fine. However, if your spouse is pushing you to have this procedure to fulfill *his* fantasies, you might want to think a little bit longer before scheduling an operation.

Some of the most successful plastic surgery procedures, as viewed through the eyes of the surgeon, have resulted in disastrous failures for the patient. This has nothing to do with the operation itself, but it has everything to do with motive and expectation. With a healthy motive and realistic expectations, you will maximize your benefits and increase your chances for success and satisfaction.

A member of the chorus of a well-known opera company decided that the reason she was not being cast in featured roles was that she needed a face-lift. She told me that she had thought it all through and concluded that the director was overlooking her for more attractive, younger-looking singers. No mention was made of her vocal talent or artistic ability.

She was furious when I told her that surgery was not the best course for her to take. Having dramatic improvement in her appearance through a face-lift would *still* not guarantee her career advancement. And, if she remained in the chorus, she would undoubtedly shift the blame from needing a face-lift to the surgeon who did a "bad" job.

The effects of plastic surgery are *permanent* in that, while the results may not last forever, the operation can never be completely undone. Therefore, think things through *before* you proceed with any plastic surgery.

Are You a Good Candidate for Plastic Surgery?

Once you have decided that you want to have plastic surgery for all the right reasons, you must determine if you are a good candidate for plastic surgery. There is more involved than wanting to have something corrected or changed beyond having the money to spend on plastic surgery and the time needed for recovery.

Two types of people who are good candidates for plastic surgery are:

* People with a strong self-image, despite the imperfection that they'd like to change.

* People who have a cosmetic flaw or physical defect that has eroded their self-esteem over time.

After an operation, the former are usually immediately pleased with the results and maintain their positive image. The latter usually require a longer period of adjustment to restore their self-esteem.

Inappropriate candidates for plastic surgery fit into six categories:

* People in crisis. Anyone going through a divorce, the death of a loved one, the loss of a job, or any number of situations must first work through the crisis before making any decision as major as undergoing plastic surgery.

* Impossible-to-please people. Those who shop around for a plastic surgeon until they get the answers they want to hear are often in search of a cure to a problem that is not primarily, if at all, physical.

* People with unrealistic expectations. These patients want to be restored to their original "perfection" after an accident or wish to turn back time to their glorious youth. Others want a celebrity's features in hopes of acquiring all that goes with stardom.

* People who are obsessed with every little flaw and believe that, once it is fixed, life will be perfect. Perfectionists may be suitable candidates for plastic surgery, but only if they understand that surgical results may not match their goals.

* People with mental illness. Anyone exhibiting delusional or paranoid behavior is a poor candidate for surgery.

+ People who smoke. Risk for every complication from breathing difficulties, skin loss, poor scarring, infection, etc., is considerably higher for smokers than nonsmokers. It cannot be emphasized enough that patients who smoke put themselves at a greater risk of developing complications than their nonsmoking counterparts. Some plastic surgeons, myself included, will refuse to perform certain operations, such as face-lifts, on patients who continue to smoke.

What You Need to Know About Risks

While precautions are taken at every turn to minimize risks, *every* aspect of medicine and surgery involves some degree of risk to the patient. The important question for you to ask is not *whether* there is any risk involved in having a particular procedure but rather what is the *degree* of risk involved. Weighing your exposure to these risks against the anticipated benefits of the procedure will help you determine whether to proceed with a proposed plan of treatment or not.

There are three general areas of risk inherent in any surgical procedure. While it is unlikely that any of them will occur, you need to know what your risks are. It does not matter whether you are talking about a gynecologic procedure, a dental procedure, a plastic surgical procedure, or any other kind of operation.

+ *Reaction to the Anesthetic:* Anesthetics, be they general, local, or local with sedation, are powerful drugs that make it possible for surgeons to do all of the things they can do today. However, there can be some unwanted side effects in their use, ranging from simple nausea to life-threatening changes in heart rhythm. There is also a potential for a serious reaction when the anesthetic your doctor uses during your operation interacts unfavorably with other medications you may be taking or other medical conditions you may have. This is the main reason that it is essential for you to give your doctor a detailed, truthful medical history. Doctors make no value judgment; they need this information.

❖ *Bleeding:* A certain amount of bleeding is expected with any surgical procedure. In its simplest form, bleeding under the skin accounts for the bruising or black-and-blue marks that appear after an operation. This aftereffect is self-limiting and does not usually represent a problem. However, excess bleeding under the skin can lead to accumulations of blood that may require secondary procedures to drain. This may compromise the outcome of the operation. Catastrophic bleeding, virtually unheard of today, can lead to vascular collapse. Again, your medical history must include any medications you take that may affect your blood clotting abilities.

❖ *Infection:* The likelihood of developing an infection varies with the type of operation being performed. In recent decades, antibiotics are frequently prescribed as a preventive measure before, during, and for a short time after an operation. This has greatly reduced the incidences of postoperative infections, but has not totally eliminated the risk. Patients taking certain medications such as steroids or who have certain medical conditions such as vascular disease, or patients who smoke, are all at higher risk of developing an infection.

What Your Doctor Needs to Know About You

Even if you just want a face-lift, your plastic surgeon wants to know about your high blood pressure. Plastic surgery is *surgery.* Your primary care physician or cardiologist may be in charge of treating your blood pressure, but your plastic surgeon is being asked to treat part of the same body that has this high blood pressure.

At your first visit, you may be surprised that your plastic surgeon wants to know so much about you: your health history, lifestyle, and emotional state, not to mention your expectations and your motives. This profile will give your surgeon information that is vital to formulating your treatment plan.

During the course of giving this health profile to your doctor, you will also have the opportunity to ask specific questions about the procedure as it relates to your current health status:

* Will my having _____ (fill in the blank: high blood pressure, diabetes, etc.) affect my having a plastic surgery operation?

* If I am diabetic, can I have a face-lift?

* If I am taking medication to control high blood pressure, can I still have a tummy tuck?

* Do I have to stop taking an antidepressant in order to have liposuction?

This is not the time to edit your health history.

There is no such thing as useless medical history. Do not withhold information *for any reason*. Some patients are embarrassed that they take antidepressants. Others fear that their surgeon may not take them seriously if they admit that they use holistic medicines on a regular basis. This information is important.

Something as simple as taking an aspirin a day may affect your operation. Aspirin, which is often taken to retard cardiovascular disease, has blood-thinning qualities that can contribute to bleeding. Your doctor also needs to know if you use nicotine gum or a patch in an effort to stop smoking. These seemingly mundane things could affect your course of treatment and recovery. Just because medications are over-the-counter does not make them harmless.

Also, answer the questions about prior operations as accurately as possible. It is essential that your doctor knows not only what might have been done but also if you had any problems with the procedure or, more specifically, with the anesthetic. Knowing this could save you from unpleasant drug or anesthetic reactions. You don't have to have an allergy to warrant avoiding certain medications. Sometimes the doctor can prescribe an alternative. If your doctor knows that a certain drug nauseates you, this unpleasant side effect can often be avoided by a substitute drug or by prescribing something to treat the nausea.

When discussing reactions to medication that you have taken in the past, you must not confuse *allergic reactions* with *side effects*. Most pain medication causes some degree of dizziness or light-headedness. This is a side effect, not an allergy. Prolonged antibiotic use may lead to a yeast infection; this, too, is a side effect, not an allergy. Many medications, taken on an empty stomach, will cause nausea. Again, this is a side effect, not an allergy.

Allergic reactions, on the other hand, usually involve development of rashes, redness, itching, welts, difficulty breathing, irregularities of heartbeat, and the like. If you are unsure whether a reaction you've had in the past is an allergy or not, assume that it is.

COMMON MEDICATIONS THAT MAY AFFECT YOUR OPERATION

- Aspirin
- Birth control pills
- Diuretics
- Weight-loss or diet pills
- Sleeping pills
- Antidepressants
- Anti-inflammatory medications, including ibuprofen

- Steroids
- Laxatives
- Homeopathic or herbal medicines; home remedies
- Megadoses of vitamins and food supplements
- Nicotine gum or patches
- Hormone patches
- Nasal sprays
- Eye drops

About Alcohol

You must also make your surgeon aware of your drinking habits. Alcohol tends to be dehydrating to the entire body, not just the skin, and is even considered to be aging to the skin. Alcohol consumption should be curtailed while you are taking pain medications as the power of the drug may be potentiated or increased.

Likewise, alcohol must never be consumed when you are taking antibiotics or any other prescription drugs.

I ask everyone who comes into my office for a consultation to complete the following questionnaire before we meet. No doubt your doctor will have his or her own version, but you might want to complete this one and take it with you for reference when you have your initial consultation.

PATIENT'S NAME: _____

Please answer the following questions carefully and thoroughly. We need this information to assure that you are given the proper drugs and medications before, during, and after your operation.

1. Do you have any medical or health problems that you are aware of? If so, please list:

   _____

   _____

2. List ANY operations, including previous plastic surgeries:

   _____

   _____

3. Have you been hospitalized in the past? ❏ Yes ❏ No

   If so, for what reasons?

   _____

   _____

4. Do you take any medications? ❏ Yes ❏ No

   If so, please list: (Include birth control pills, sleeping pills, anti-depressants, aspirin, Advil, Nuprin, Motrin, ibuprofen, vitamins, food supplements, and laxatives.)

   _____

5. Do you smoke? ❏ Yes ❏ No

   If so, how much and for how long?

   _____

6. Do you drink alcoholic beverages? ❏ Yes ❏ No

   If so, how much and for how long?

   _____

7. Do you take or use any recreational drugs, such as marijuana, Quaaludes, cocaine, or other drugs? NOTE: Failure to answer these questions *honestly* can result in serious problems during surgery. Use of street drugs and some tranquilizers, combined with medication used in surgery, can be lethal. Any and all drug use should be discussed with the doctor. All answers are kept strictly confidential.

_____

_____

8. Are you allergic to or have you had any problems with medications or anesthetics?   ❏ Yes   ❏ No

   If so, please describe:

_____

_____

9. Does anyone in your family have a history of allergies or problems with anesthetics?   ❏ Yes   ❏ No

   If so, please describe:

_____

10. Do you have or have you had:

a. High or low blood pressure   ❏ Yes   ❏ No

b. Heart disease or chest pain   ❏ Yes   ❏ No

c. Lung problems or asthma   ❏ Yes   ❏ No

d. Diabetes or high or low blood sugar   ❏ Yes   ❏ No

e. Stomach problems, ulcers, or gastritis   ❏ Yes   ❏ No

f. Liver disease or hepatitis   ❏ Yes   ❏ No

g. Kidney disease   ❏ Yes   ❏ No

h. Thyroid disease   ❏ Yes   ❏ No

i. Anemia or problems with blood clotting ❑ Yes   ❑ No

j. Varicose veins, phlebitis (inflamed veins), blood clots in your legs ❑ Yes   ❑ No

k. Seizures, convulsions, or fainting spells ❑ Yes   ❑ No

l. AIDS, ARC, or positive HIV blood test ❑ Yes   ❑ No

11. Do you have any loose or capped teeth or dentures? ❑ Yes   ❑ No

12. What is your height? _____ Weight? _____ Age? _____ Sex?

13. Is there any possibility that you might be pregnant? ❑ Yes   ❑ No

PLEASE NOTE: Pregnant women should *not* have anesthesia. The drugs used in surgery and anesthesia can harm the fetus and cause birth defects. If there is any possibility that you might be pregnant, you must see your family physician or gynecologist to exclude this possibility *before* having any surgery or anesthesia.

I certify that the above is true and correct to the best of my knowledge.

_____   _____

NAME   DATE

_____

SIGNATURE

Would you like a third party present during your examination? ❑ Yes   ❑ No

I include the final question for two reasons. The first is for your comfort. Some people feel more at ease if there is a friend or spouse, or even a nurse, in the room during an examination. The second reason may be less obvious: Four ears are better than two. Your partner will be able to take notes for you or help you remember what was discussed.

Additional Helpful Information

Doctors need to know more than just your name and what you want done before we can treat you. After all, you *are* contemplating having an operation and, while it may be cosmetic and may be performed as an outpatient procedure in your doctor's office during your lunch hour, it is still an operation with risks. The information that you provide will help to identify these risk factors so that they can be more easily managed.

I realize that you are my patient, and, while it is you who is having something done, this may also affect others in your life, especially your spouse or significant other. The more information you share, the more these people can be involved in your experience.

Early in my practice, a woman came to me for a face-lift. On the day of her operation, she told her husband to pick her up at an appointed time. When he arrived, he was surprised to find out that she had had *any* operation, never mind a face-lift! He was totally unprepared for the role of caregiver he was asked to play. It took considerable time to calm him down, reassure him that his wife was just fine, and then instruct him on what needed to be done over the course of the next several days. In effect, one patient turned into two.

I have since changed our office policy, insisting that patients let me know in advance who will be caring for them and provide written instructions for postoperative care to that individual.

This information requested in this sample is pretty standard—everyday things, like address, phone numbers, and social security number, that you probably won't need to think about. However, I've included the sample questionnaire to make sure that you have all the information ready.

ABOUT YOU

Today's Date: _____

Name: _____

What you prefer
to be called: _____

Date of birth: _____ Age: _____

❑ Single   ❑ Married   ❑ Divorced   ❑ Widowed   ❑ Separated

Social Security #: _____

Home Address: _____

Home Phone: _____

Other Phone: _____

EMPLOYER INFORMATION

Employer's Name: _____

Address: _____

Work Phone: _____ Ext.: _____

What you do there: _____

Referred by: _____

SPOUSE INFORMATION

Name: _____

Home Phone: _____

Employer: _____

Work Phone: _____

Social Security #: _____

Date of birth: _____

Don't Keep Your Operation Secret

The necessity of an emergency contact name and number is self-evident. Just make sure that the person you list is aware that you are having an operation and will be available at that time if needed.

IN EVENT OF AN EMERGENCY WHO SHOULD WE CONTACT?

Name: _____

Relationship: _____

Day Phone: _____

Home Phone: _____

How to Find the Right Surgeon

A savvy professional woman told me of a consultation she had with a plastic surgeon who has a long list of prominent patients. She arrived at his office slightly before the appointed time and was kept waiting for an hour and a half before "being received" by the doctor. After her "audience" with the doctor, which lasted for only twelve minutes, she was ushered out, thinking she would be taken in for a more complete examination by the doctor. Instead, she was asked to fill out a statement of full financial disclosure, more detailed than that required by her co-op board. She respectfully declined and left. "Then he sent me a bill for $1,500!"

A young man came to me to have plastic surgery to correct work that had been done on his prominent ears. He learned too late—after the operation—that the "plastic surgeon" who performed that procedure specialized in *pediatrics*.

One young man in his mid-twenties found his way to my office after consulting at least a half dozen other plastic surgeons. His face was riddled with acne scars. He also had a prominent nose. He told me, up front, that he wanted to have his acne scars treated. Why hadn't he chosen one of the previous surgeons he had consulted? He wanted his *acne scars* repaired, but every other doctor he had seen wanted to "fix" his nose. They hadn't listened to him. Yes, his nose was large, just like almost everyone else in his family. His primary concern was his pocked skin.

Obviously, finding the *right* plastic surgeon is more involved than checking the Yellow Pages under "Plastic Surgeons" or responding to an advertisement. You can't even tell how good or even how reputable a doctor is by the address, fee schedules, media attention, or roster of celebrity clients.

Begin your search for the right plastic surgeon by collecting names of prospective candidates. Good resources include:

- *Friends*. Ask anyone you know who's had a procedure like the one you're considering. Ask how they were treated by the doctor and his staff. Are they pleased with the results? How long was their recuperation? (Don't pick a surgeon on *one* person's recommendation. Every patient is unique; so is every surgery. Your experience may be quite different from your friend's.)

- *Doctors*. Ask your family doctor for a referral. How many patients has he or she referred to this plastic surgeon? Would the doctor send a family member to this plastic surgeon?

- *Nurses*. An operating room nurse is a great source of information about plastic surgeons. If you know one, or know someone who knows one, set up a meeting. You'll probably get a valuable assessment of a surgeon's work.

❖ *Hospitals.* Call your community medical center and ask for the names of the *board-certified* plastic surgeons on staff. Be sure to ask the names of doctors who had official approval to do the particular operation you are considering.

❖ *The American Society of Plastic and Reconstructive Surgeons (ASPRS).* This association of board-certified plastic surgeons offers The Plastic Surgery Information Center to answer consumer questions. Call the toll-free number, 1-800-635-0635, and leave your name, address, and the procedure you're considering. The association will give you the names of five member plastic surgeons in your area who regularly perform that procedure. Membership in the ASPRS is open only to doctors certified by the American Board of Plastic Surgery (ABPS).

Checking Credentials

Once you've compiled a list of prospects, start checking their credentials. Good credentials won't guarantee you a successful outcome, but they can increase the odds in your favor.

❖ Is the doctor *board certified?* If so, by whom? While it is not the only certifying board, the American Board of Plastic Surgery (ABPS) is the benchmark for certifications, defining the standards within the field. ABPS certification guarantees that this doctor was graduated from an accredited medical school, *plus* at least five years of residency training, usually three years of general surgery plus two years of plastic surgery. Before applying, a doctor must practice plastic surgery for two years and pass comprehensive oral and written exams.

Another reputable certifying body for plastic surgeons is the American Association of Aesthetic Surgeons.

You should also be aware that some dermatologists and ear-nose-throat specialists often perform plastic surgery procedures and may be qualified in a specific area of plastic surgery. I say this not to imply that they are not capable of performing plastic surgery but to explain that they are *not* board certified in **plastic and reconstructive surgery.** (Personally, if a doctor I am considering for a reconstructive or plastic surgery procedure is *not* a board certified plastic surgeon, I would definitely want to know what his or her specialty and certification are.)

❖ Where was the doctor trained? Has the surgeon completed an accredited residency program specifically in plastic surgery at a hospital with strong plastic and reconstructive surgery training? Such a program should include two or three years of intensive training that concentrates on the full spectrum of reconstructive and cosmetic procedures.

❖ What are the doctor's professional affiliations? As with board certification, some professional societies have more prestige than others. If a surgeon says he or she belongs to a specific society, get the exact name. You can call the society and find out what the membership requirements are and then verify the doctor's membership. The American Society of Plastic and Reconstructive Surgeons (ASPRS) is one of the largest organizations representing plastic and reconstructive surgeons. In addition to requiring certification by the American Board of Plastic Surgeons, members are subject to peer review, must participate in continuing medical education, and must adhere to a stringent code of ethics.

❖ Where does your doctor have hospital privileges? Even if your operation will be performed in the doctor's own surgical facility, the doctor should also have privileges to perform *that* procedure in an accredited medical facility in your community. This means the surgeon is subject to review by a body of his or her peers. Call the hospital to verify any affiliations.

♦ While there is no magic number of years in practice or procedures performed to measure experience, you should be satisfied that the plastic surgeon you choose is both well versed in the procedure you're having and up to date on all aspects of this surgery. Two good questions to ask: How often do you perform this procedure? When was the last time you did it?

Once you narrow down your list to two or three surgeons, make an appointment for a preliminary consultation. You will, in all probability, be charged for these appointments, whether or not you choose one of these surgeons. It will, however, be money well spent.

This will give you an opportunity to compare the doctors' personalities and doctor-patient manner. Observe how the doctors treat their staffs and how these staffs treat you and other patients in the waiting room. Find out about fees, and get their opinion on the type of surgery you want to have. Make note of how openly they answer your questions and how forthcoming they are in explaining the risks involved.

I suggest that you write down your questions beforehand to make sure you don't leave anything out, and write down the surgeon's responses. These questions should be answered clearly and thoroughly in language that you understand.

What to Expect from Your Initial Consultation

How you are treated in the course of making your appointment may give you a sense of how everything else will go.

Use your time in the waiting room to review any biographical material provided by the doctor. Also talk with staff and other patients. Many but not all patients may feel comfortable about talking with others about their experience. Regardless of the procedure, such small talk will give you a good sense of how patients are cared for by this doctor and staff. Not everyone will want to open up, but you may be able to find someone willing to speak candidly.

Here are some general things to be on the lookout for in this interview/consultation:

* Are you treated with courtesy? Are you listened to? Do you and the doctor have a mutual understanding of why you are considering plastic surgery and what plastic surgery you want?

* Are you asked about your motivations and expectations? Did the doctor discuss them with you and solicit your reactions to their recommendations? Are you encouraged to ask questions and speak freely? As the patient, you must be a participant in your care.

* Does the doctor offer alternatives, where appropriate, without pressuring you to consider unnecessary or additional procedures? If a doctor attempts to steer you into additional plastic surgery or appears to have an agenda of his or her own, you might want to keep looking.

* Does the surgeon explain any risks in the operation you want to have as well as any possible variations in outcome? Ask about risks and variations yourself, should this information not be volunteered by the doctor. You need to know the *worst-case* scenarios rather than just the best. You can't go by tabloid TV and stories in popular magazines. If a doctor shows you a scrapbook of photographs of patients or uses computer imaging to show you possible results, promising that you'll have the same outcome,

keep looking. Human tissue doesn't perform the same way as an image on a computer screen.

Don't be afraid to ask a doctor questions. If an answer isn't clear, keep asking until you get an answer that you understand. It may not necessarily be the answer you want to hear. Make sure that you get *your* questions answered clearly. Getting the information you need will diffuse much of the anxiety and fear you may have.

❖ Is the doctor willing to answer all questions about professional qualifications and experience? Are you given a complete breakdown of costs and payment policies?

Full disclosure is your right as a consumer. Any lack of clarity about a doctor's background or fees may be indicative of other areas of lax communication.

What If Things Go "Wrong"?

No one approaches plastic surgery with the expectation that they will be made worse instead of better. It is a reality that medicine is an imperfect science. Plastic surgery is no exception.

It is for this reason that you should discuss with your doctor not only the expected outcome of a given procedure but also the unexpected. While precautions are taken at every step to avoid complications that might compromise results, they sometimes happen.

Fortunately, virtually every unfavorable result can be improved, either by the passage of time or by a second procedure. In the event that time does not heal everything, and you do require a second procedure, you will want to know what additional expenses might be incurred. There is no set policy in this regard. Some surgeons perform corrective secondary procedures at no charge, others reduce their fees, and others make no fee adjustments.

Although you are unlikely to face this situation, you would be wise to address this possibility—however remote—*before* undertaking any procedure. Determine your surgeon's policy regarding secondary procedures and factor this into your decision making.

When it comes to the selection of a plastic surgeon, the final decision is yours.

Checklist for the Plastic Surgery Consumer

GOOD BET

- ❑ Recommended by a friend who had a similar procedure

- ❑ Recommended by family doctor or operating room nurse

- ❑ Board certified by the American Board of Plastic Surgery

- ❑ Member of American Society of Plastic and Reconstructive Surgery and other specialized professional associations

- ❑ Has privileges to do your procedure at an accredited hospital

- ❑ Completed residency in a specialty related to your procedure: plastic surgery (all procedures); dermatology (skin); otolaryngology (head and neck); orthopedic (hand or limb reconstruction)

NEED MORE INFORMATION

- ❑ Got name from telephone directory or other advertisement

- ❑ Saw doctor on television or other media

- ❑ General physicians referral service

- ❑ Recommended by "someone", i.э., not necessarily someone you know well and respect

KEEP LOOKING

- ❑ Certified in a specialty other than plastic surgery or related field

- ❑ Completed residency in unrelated specialty

- ❑ Does not have hospital privileges for your procedure

- ❑ Unwilling to answer your questions to *your* satisfaction

- ❑ Impatient, arrogant, even rude to you and staff; unprofessional office or personal manner

- ❑ Unwilling to be specific when discussing costs and fees

- ❑ Makes promises about results, absence of pain, etc.

- ❑ Pressures you to have additional procedures

How to Evaluate a Same-Day Surgical Facility

These days, most plastic surgery operations are performed on an ambulatory or same-day basis. This might be in an operating room in the doctor's office, a self-contained or freestanding surgical facility, or part of a hospital.

Your choice of an ambulatory or same-day surgical facility for plastic surgery is an important part of planning for your operation. Just as you must be comfortable with your surgeon and your surgeon's staff, you must feel at ease with the place where the operation will be performed.

Many plastic surgeons recommend ambulatory surgery because of the financial savings and convenience as well as the increased privacy. It also affords a level of personalized care not associated with an overnight hospital stay.

Ambulatory surgery may not be for every patient. Only you and your surgeon can decide if you are a good candidate for same-day surgery. You'll need to have someone to accompany you home and remain with you for twenty-four to forty-eight hours postoperatively as your doctor advises. If you have no one able to do this, your doctor can arrange for you to enter a postoperative recovery facility until you can care for yourself or, as another alternative, reserve a trained nurse to accompany you from the facility and then stay with you during this crucial period.

When planning surgery at an ambulatory surgical facility, ask if the facility is accredited. This will be an indication that the facility meets strict guidelines for equipment, staff, hospital access, and anesthesia administration. In addition, doctors performing surgery at the facility must have privileges to perform the same procedures at an accredited hospital.

Ask your doctor about the accreditation of the ambulatory center.

A certificate of accreditation will usually be prominently displayed in the facility. Among organizations accrediting walk-in surgical centers are:

❖ The American Association for Accreditation of Ambulatory Surgery Facilities (AAAASF)
1202 Allanson Road
Mundelein, IL 60060
847-949-6058

❖ The Accreditation Association for Ambulatory Health Care (AAAHC)
9933 Lawler Avenue
Skokie, IL 60077
847-676-9610

❖ The Joint Commission on Accreditation of Healthcare Organizations (JCAHO)
1 Renaissance Boulevard
Oakbrook Terrace, IL 60181
630-916-5600

The American Society of Plastic and Reconstructive Surgeons can tell you if a plastic surgeon's facility is accredited.

AAAASF inspects only ambulatory plastic surgery centers. This is a not-for-profit association that inspects member facilities, measuring patient care, quality, and safety against rigorous standards. Certification requires yearly self-examination with recertification inspection by the association every three years.

This association classifies ambulatory facilities as A, B, or C. In A facilities, procedures are performed under local anesthesia. In B and C facilities, medications to relieve tension or tranquilizers may be given before anesthesia is administered. Local anesthesia with sedation may be used during the operation only in B and C facilities.

Most operations are performed in centers classified as B or C. Standards vary slightly between the two. Both have life-support equipment, just as a hospital operating room. In Class B facilities, intravenous sedation may be administered, while Class C facilities are authorized to administer general anesthesia.

Fees charged by ambulatory facilities are usually based on the procedures performed at the center.

Fees and What You Need to Know About Insurance

This section addresses several points. First is the payment schedule. This, of course, varies from doctor to doctor, but most require payment in advance for procedures that are not covered by insurance.

In the event that your operation *may* be covered by insurance, you and your doctor may arrange for a full or partial advance payment plan. **This needs to be resolved before any procedure is performed.** Just remember: It's *your* responsibility to see to it that your insurance company pays your doctor, not the other way around. If they do not pay, then you are ultimately liable for these costs unless the doctor participates in your health maintenance organization.

There are three components to the cost of your plastic surgery. Do not assume that the surgeon's fee automatically includes the others.

❖ *The Surgeon's Fee:* This is the fee charged by the surgeon to perform your operation, and it may also include the fee for any surgical assistant, if required.

❖ *Anesthesia Fee:* This fee is charged for the administration of anesthesia by an anesthesiologist, an anesthetist (usually a nurse trained in administering anesthesia), or by the surgeon.

❖ *Facility Fee:* Depending upon where your operation is performed, there may be a separate charge for the use of the operating facility.

Usually, once your insurance considers a procedure to be covered by your policy, this coverage applies to all three fees.

Your consent is required for taking pre- and postoperative photographs. These are necessary to your course of treatment and become a part of your medical record. These pictures may be taken by the doctor or by a professional medical photographer. Any concerns you have about confidentiality and use of these pictures should be discussed with your doctor during your initial consultation.

IMPORTANT INFORMATION

We invite you to discuss frankly with us any questions regarding our services. The best medical service is based on a friendly, mutual understanding between physician and patient.

Our office policy requires payment in full for all medical services rendered at the time of visit unless other arrangements have been made with the business manager. If the account is not paid within ninety days of the date of service and no financial arrangement has been made, you will be responsible for any expenses incurred in collecting your account.

I hereby authorize payment of medical benefits directly to the physician of benefits due me for services rendered. I further authorize the physician and/or supplier to release any information required to process insurance claims.

I also hereby consent to the taking of preoperative and postoperative photographs of the operative area(s) and to their subsequent utilization for medical and instructional purposes as deemed necessary.

I understand the above information and guarantee this form was completed correctly to the best of my knowledge and understand it is my responsibility to inform this office of any changes in my medical status.

_____

SIGNATURE OF RESPONSIBLE PERSON   DATE

Perhaps the most self-explanatory part of this preliminary process is providing account information. As you will see, this is where your doctor will ask who is ultimately responsible for your account and how it will be paid.

ACCOUNT INFORMATION
_____

Person Ultimately Responsible for Account

            Name: _____

    Relationship: _____

Billing Address: _____

                 _____

Social Security #: _____

Employer: _____

Day Phone: _____ Ext.: _____

Desired Method of Payment

❏ Cash   ❏ Check   ❏ Credit Card #_____

Expiration Date: _____

Insurance: What's Covered

In today's climate, most if not all cosmetic procedures performed to reshape normal body parts in order to improve the patient's appearance and self-esteem are **not** covered by insurance. Only reconstructive procedures that treat congenital defects, developmental anomalies, injury, or some *functional* problem are routinely covered by most policies.

The gray areas in coverage for plastic surgery require special consideration. This usually involves operations that may be reconstructive or cosmetic, depending on a specific patient's condition. For example, an upper blepharoplasty—eyelid lift—is a procedure normally performed for cosmetic improvement; however, if the eyelids are drooping sufficiently to obscure a patient's vision, the operation may be considered reconstructive and, consequently, worthy of full or partial coverage. Even rhinoplasty—nose surgery—may be covered if the surgery will correct a defect that causes breathing difficulty.

Insurance carriers look at the *primary* reason for your operation. They will ask if the operation is being performed to provide relief of symptoms or for cosmetic or aesthetic improvement.

To make sure you receive the maximum reimbursement you deserve—especially if you are electing to have a surgery that could be construed as cosmetic *or* reconstructive—ask your primary care physician to provide you with documentation of your need for this procedure. This must be done *in advance* of your operation.

While doctors can almost certainly say what is *not* covered, often they can not say specifically what *is*. Beware of the doctor who offers to "doctor" your insurance forms to get paid for a procedure. A doctor who will lie to your insurer will almost surely lie to you.

Coverage varies from one company to another, so you must check with your individual carrier.

Understanding Your Medical Insurance

Pull out that copy of your medical insurance policy and take a close look at what it says about what *is* and what *is not* covered and how much coverage will be provided. Read your policy and benefits manual carefully. If you have any questions, you may want to discuss your plans for plastic surgery with your insurance plan manager.

Three common cost-sharing options are:

◆ A *deductible* requires that a certain amount of medical expenses be paid by the patient before the insurance company begins paying coverage. Standard deductibles are $100, $200, or $500. After this amount is met, the insurer will begin paying, according to the terms of the policy— 75 to 80 percent of covered medical costs. You, the patient, will be responsible for any remaining balance.

◆ A *flat-rate co-payment* calls for the patient to pay a defined share of covered medical costs, based on the policy. The insurance company is responsible for the balance.

◆ A *percentage-based co-payment* requires the patient to pay a percentage of covered medical costs with the insurer paying the balance or a fixed amount based on the policy.

There are numerous co-payment arrangements that include deductibles and fees. Your benefits coordinator or insurance representative will be able to explain the fine points for you. Make sure that you understand every point of coverage before having surgery.

Insurance Glossary for the Patient Considering Plastic Surgery

Some terms you may come across in your request for insurance coverage of your plastic surgery include:

Co-payment   The portion of covered costs paid by the patient. Typically, this amount will be based on a percentage or flat rate.

Coordination of benefits   Occurs when a patient is eligible for coverage by more than one insurance carrier. Benefits of the plans are coordinated so that a patient may receive maximum benefits.

CPT code   A number used to identify medical services. CPT stands for *current procedural terminology,* a system developed by the American Medical Association. Physicians use codes in billing for services.

Deductible   The total amount of covered medical care costs that must be paid by the patient before the insurance carrier begins paying or reimbursing payment of benefits.

Exclusion   A condition or circumstance not covered by insurance.

ICD-9 code   The international classification of disease code, used to indicate the diagnosis—illness, disease, or trauma—for which care is given. CPT and ICD-9 codes must correlate correctly for an insurance carrier to consider payment.

Preauthorization letter A letter written by a physician to an insurance company prior to surgery, explaining the procedure in detail and requesting confirmation that the patient is covered, that planned services are covered, and the level of coverage.

Predetermination A review process conducted by an insurance carrier to verify medical necessity of an operation or treatment. Often this is a condition of payment by a carrier.

Insurance

Here's what I ask my patients about insurance. You may want to have all this information ready to give your doctor.

PRIMARY INSURANCE COMPANY

Company Name: _____

Address: _____

Phone #: _____

Group # (Plan, Local, or Policy #): _____

Insured's Name: _____

Relationship: _____

Date of Birth: _____

Social Security #: _____

Insured's Employer: _____

SECONDARY INSURANCE COMPANY

Company Name: _____

Address: _____

Phone #: _____

Group # (Plan, Local, or Policy #): _____

Insured's Name: _____

Relationship: _____

Date of Birth: _____

Social Security #: _____

Insured's Employer: _____

Your Guide to
Plastic Surgery Procedures

~

What You **Should** Know

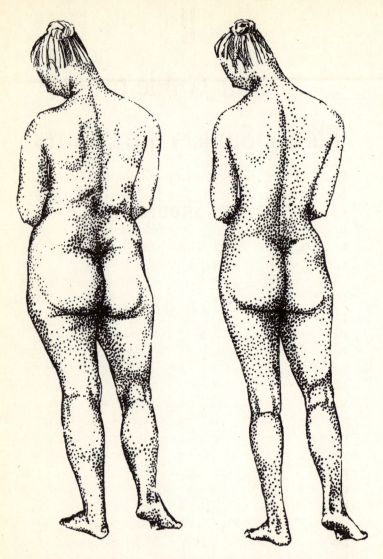

Liposuction: The before and after figures show how liposuction can be used to contour the body.

1

Liposuction

~

Betty, in her mid-thirties, is five feet, six inches tall, healthy, and fit. She has a high-pressure Wall Street job, where she'd grown accustomed to being treated like one of the boys. She may not mind being treated like one of the boys, but she didn't want to carry the potbelly that so many of her male coworkers sported.

Despite faithful workouts at her local gym, she couldn't trim her abs. In fact, she was frequently asked if she was pregnant. Betty had a genetic predisposition to fat deposits in her abdomen. Normal diet and exercise would never get rid of this pouch of fat cells.

Betty sought my services for *limited liposuction* of her lower abdomen, a procedure that would not interfere with her frenetic work schedule and did not require that she be put to sleep. I assured her that she would be out of her office no more than a long lunch hour and that she would be fully conscious throughout the procedure. She arrived for her appointment at one P.M. She was on the operating table for no more than forty-five minutes and back at her desk by three P.M.

Betty's postoperative swelling was the same size as her preprocedure tummy, so there was no visible difference in her figure at this time. None of her colleagues noticed a thing when she went back to work on the day of her procedure and in the days to follow.

After about six weeks, the swelling was gone completely.

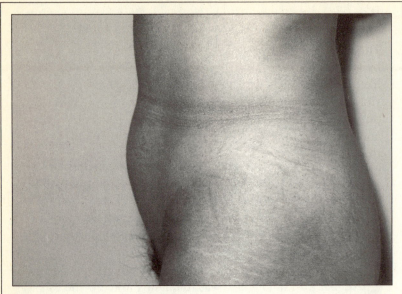

Limited Liposuction: Before and approximately six weeks after limited liposuction of the lower abdomen.

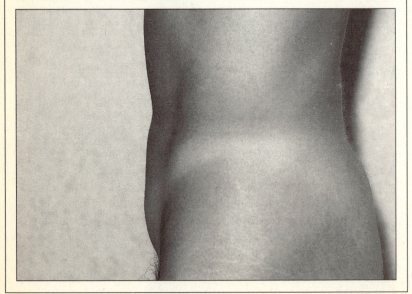

It's a Matter of Fat

The *number* of fat cells in the body is, as a rule, established by the time we reach puberty, if not before. These cells are like balloons, with an amazing capacity of expansion and storage of fat. When we're "too fat," these cells are, simply put, inflated. To slim and firm the body, eat a balanced diet and have an exercise program that includes aerobic exercise to burn calories, stretches for flexibility and weight maintenanace, and isometric training to build and tone muscles.

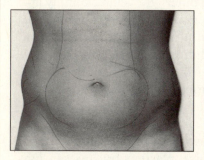
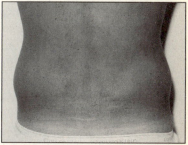

Preoperative views of a 33-year-old male patient showing the common "spare tire" or "love handles." The faint lines (left) are preoperative markings drawn by the surgeon to outline the areas being tested.

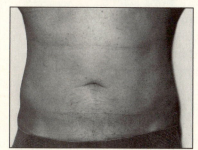
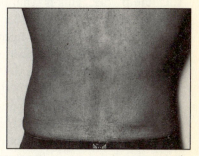

Six weeks after liposuction, while considerable skin contraction has occurred, note that minor irregularities are still visible. Swelling will not be fully resolved for three months.

Fat weighs little, relative to the space it occupies. A pound of fat takes up a lot more room than a pound of muscle or bone.

For many, all the exercise and careful eating in the world still leaves them with pockets of stubborn fat. Spot reduction exercises are of limited, if any, value. Some people simply lack the genetic tools to achieve the body they want.

Lipectomy and liposuction are procedures to modify volume and contour, neither is meant to be a method of **weight** reduction.

Once exercise, dieting, not to mention carefully selected clothing—undergarments *and* outerwear—and skillfully applied cosmetics can no longer support the *illusion* of the body of your dreams, you can turn to plastic surgery for a conditionally permanent solution. Liposuction does not give you permission to sit in front of the TV all day or pig out at the buffet and expect to keep your new, shapely figure. You still need to maintain a healthy diet and exercise regimen.

Just as an artist chisels away excess marble or molds and shapes clay to form a sculpture, plastic surgeons can use their skills to remove excess fat to reshape the body. But, the body is not as predictable as stone or clay in its response to this handiwork. This is where art meets science.

Until the mid to late 1980s, surgical body contouring was accomplished by *dermato lipectomy*, surgical removal of fat and skin. This will be explained in the next chapter. Still effectively used in areas like the abdomen, where muscles and skin have been so stretched by massive fluctuations in weight that they can't return to normal, dermato lipectomy has been replaced by a simpler, less invasive body contouring procedure, most commonly called *liposuction*, more formally, *suction assisted lipectomy*.

Today, liposuction is the most requested plastic surgery procedure in the country, according to American Society of Plastic and Reconstructive Surgeons statistics.

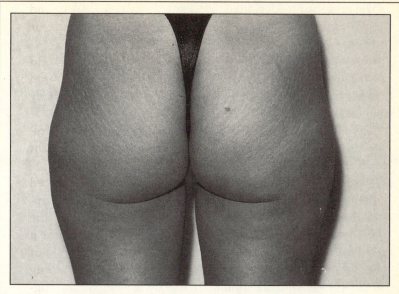

Liposuction of the thighs: Note that incisions, placed in the buttocks creases, are not visible two months postoperatively.

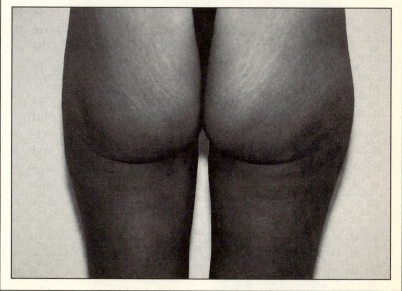

Overview

Ideal candidates for liposuction, which may be performed on virtually any part of the body, are close to their normal weight and have good skin tone. These patients have pockets of fat in specific areas of the body that are resistant to diet and exercise. Although many patients don't fall into this ideal, they can still benefit greatly from this procedure, as long as they are realistic in their expectations.

Women commonly request liposuction on their hips (see page 41), abdomens, and thighs, as well as knees, calves, and ankles. Men generally want help with their waists and abdomens (love handles and spare tires, see page 39). Both sexes want their double chins and jowls treated (see pages 50 and 51). Liposuction may also be effective in reducing enlarged male breasts, a condition known as gynecomastia (see page 189).

Liposuction can be performed on virtually any part of the body—abdomen and flanks, ankles, arms, buttocks, calves,

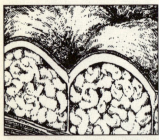
Cellulite, shown in this drawing, is a non-medical term used to describe fatty deposits that give the skin an uneven, irregular texture.

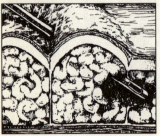
In liposuction, a canula is used to remove excess fat while breaking the skin bands that connect skin to muscle tissue in the area being treated.

chest, chin and jawline, knees, and even the inner and outer thighs. Limited or spot liposuction is ideal for patients who have small, localized problem areas, and standard liposuction is designed to treat larger areas, such as the entire abdomen or buttocks.

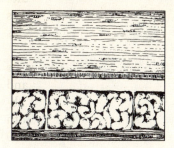

After liposuction, new bands form and the skin contracts to give a tauter, smoother skin surface.

Definitions

Canula   A small, hollow tube. In liposuction, it is inserted into the skin through one or more tiny incisions near the area to be suctioned. Attached to a syringe or vacuum pressure unit, the canula is guided by the surgeon to aspirate unwanted fat.

Cellulite   A nonmedical term used to describe fatty deposits that give the skin an uneven, dimpled texture.

Laser liposuction   A developing technology that uses light energy to break up fat for removal.

Limited liposuction   Also called spot or lunch hour liposuction. Small, specific fatty areas are treated, removing one to two cups of fat. This procedure does not involve tightening of muscles or skin resection.

Standard liposuction   Liposuction treatment of a larger area, such as the abdomen, or buttocks and thighs, removing one to two liters of fat. This does not involve tightening of muscles or skin resection.

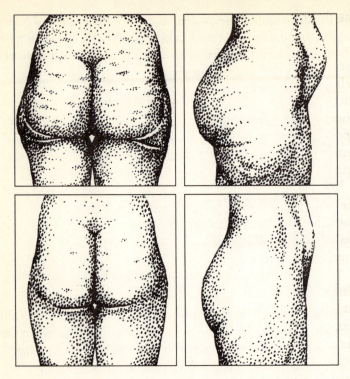

Back and side views, before and after liposuction.

Tumescent/tumescence   A liposuction technique that introduces large amounts of dilute anesthetic solution into the area to be treated. The fluid causes the area to balloon, ensuring minimal discomfort to the patient and making aspiration of the fat easier.

Ultrasound   A newly FDA-approved technology that utilizes sound waves applied to the skin surface to break up the fat for easier removal in a process known as ultrasound assisted liposuction (UAL).

Umbilicus   The navel.

The Procedure

In liposuction, a thin, hollow tube, or *canula*, is inserted through one or more incisions near the designated area. When a small, specific area is being treated by limited liposuction, a syringe is usually connected to the canula to produce a vacuum. A vacuum pump is used for standard liposuction when larger areas are being treated. This allows removal of the unwanted fat in the layer between skin and muscle.

Your surgeon may use a dry technique, simply suctioning the fat, or, more likely, the tumescent technique that introduces a dilute solution of anesthetic into the area, making it easier to aspirate the fat and minimizing postoperative discomfort.

Two technologies that are being applied in liposuction are ultrasound and laser. While both are receiving much media attention, neither has earned widespread acceptance. Ultrasound waves are used to liquify the fat, making aspiration easier. Laser uses light energy to the same end. Ultrasound technology is ahead of laser in development and has recently received FDA approval. Initially administered under the skin with a wandlike probe, it now is applied externally to break up fat. This liquid fat is more easily suctioned. Advocates assert that this causes less bleeding and tissue damage, making recovery easier (see chapter 11).

Length of Procedure

Limited liposuction can take forty-five minutes to an hour.

Standard liposuction takes one and a half to two hours. Multiple areas of the body may be treated at the same time.

Anesthesia

You and your doctor have several options:

Local anesthesia: An injection of anesthetic numbs the area being treated.

Local with sedation: Medication administered by vein to induce sleep followed by an injection of an anesthetic to numb the area being treated.

General anesthesia: An anesthetic gas is administered to induce sleep and a ventilator is required to assist breathing.

In almost all liposuction operations, regardless of the chosen anesthetic, your doctor will use a local anesthetic with epinephrine, a vascular constrictor, to reduce bleeding during the operation and aid in controlling postoperative pain.

In/Outpatient

Most liposuction is performed in an ambulatory surgical center on an outpatient basis. Extensive procedures may warrant a short inpatient stay.

Incisions/Scarring

You will have incisions measuring three to six millimeters where the canula was inserted. Remember that there are 25.4 millimeters to the inch. Sutures may or may not be used. Scars, though present, are usually placed where they will be most inconspicuous.

Pain

With local anesthesia alone, you will feel some vibration and friction during the procedure. You may also experience a stinging sensation as the canula is moved closer to the edges of the area that has been numbed.

Pain is described as achy-sore muscle type, like that experienced after a strenuous workout. This pain is not toothache sharp.

As a rule, pain after limited liposuction is easily managed with acetaminophen or mild pain medication. After standard liposuction, pain medication is prescribed for one to two days, followed by acetaminophen or mild pain medication. Patients often say they feel sore and bruised, but are able to tolerate it with ease.

Specific Risks

❖ Excessive blood loss can lead to shock.

❖ Fluid or blood accumulation under the skin may resolve itself spontaneously or require surgical drainage.

❖ Skin irregularities, such as dimpling, rippling, bagginess, or asymmetry are frequent but seldom permanent. If they persist, they can usually be corrected quite easily with a second limited procedure to smooth out the skin.

❖ Pigmentation changes may become permanent if the skin is exposed to the sun too soon after the operation.

Recovery Time

Return to Work
❖ Desk Job:
     Limited: You can return to work immediately.
     Standard: Give yourself three to four days to rest.
❖ Manual labor: Bending, lifting heavy weights, and straining are restricted for one week.

With a support garment, you should be increasing your activity level at a steady pace, with full return of energy and strength by six weeks. Some patients take less time when smaller areas are treated; few take longer.

Exercise

While walking is encouraged to ensure ample circulation and promote healing, strenuous exercise is avoided for the first week. Most patients can resume their usual level of aerobic activity a week after the operation, as long as a compression garment, such as Lycra workout shorts, is worn for one month.

Once bruising has disappeared, feel free to resume weight training as well.

Sex

Same as for exercise. Wait for about a week. Don't try anything new or strenuous for a couple of weeks.

Sun

Stay out of the sun for the first week. Always use sunscreen.

Travel

There are no restrictions on travel by automobile, airplane, or bus. You may not feel comfortable sitting for extended periods of time for about a week.

Frequency/Duration of Results

Results are permanent if you maintain your healthy diet and exercise regimen. If you revert to poor eating and exercise habits, you can outeat your results. You'll have fewer fat cells, but they'll be fatter.

What to Expect

Some degree of bruising can be expected during the first week to ten days. If you tend to bruise easily, expect to see a wider range of colors than someone who tends not to. *Many patients find that eating fresh pineapple during their post operative period helps to make bruising disappear faster, thanks to the presence of bromelain, an enzyme that dissolves protein.*

You can also expect swelling, which commonly peaks at three to four days and disappears within six weeks. Some patients report numbness and a burning sensation at various intervals postoperatively with symptoms dissipating within four to six weeks.

An elastic bandage, support stockings, girdle, or special support garment usually is worn nearly continuously over the area that has been suctioned for the first week following the operation. It is recommended that patients with poorer skin tone wear some type of support garment as much as possible for the month after the operation to reduce the possibility of skin dimpling, sagging, unevenness, or waviness.

If you have standard liposuction, some surgeons may insert a drainage tube beneath your skin for one to three days to remove any fluid buildup.

I often recommend that patients have medical massage therapy, sometimes called lymphatic drainage massage therapy, beginning the second or third week after their operation to relieve stiffness and promote circulation, thereby decreasing swelling. Ask your doctor if you would benefit from this treatment.

Fees/Insurance

The usual cost of liposuction is between $1,500 and $2,500 per site for limited liposuction, $3,000 to $5,000 per site for standard liposuction. (These figures do not include the cost of an appropriate compression garment.)

Liposuction is not usually covered by insurance unless it is performed as part of a medically indicated procedure.

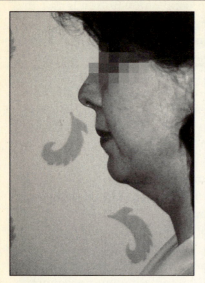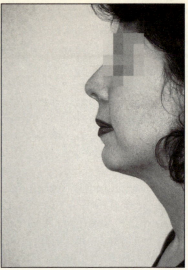

Liposuction: Before and six weeks after liposuction was performed on this patient's chin. There is little evidence of swelling. The illusion of a longer neck has been achieved.

Important Questions to Ask About Liposuction

❖ How many scars will there be?

❖ Where will the scars be? *(Ask your surgeon to draw lines or dots with a marker to show where he plans to make incisions so you can see for yourself.)*

❖ What will the skin in the treated area look like?

❖ Will I need to wear a compression garment, and what does it look like? *(Take this into consideration when scheduling your operation, especially in hot weather.)*

❖ What is a realistic recovery timetable for me?

Chin Procedure

Jane, a thirty-something career woman, had inherited her grandmother's lack of a neckline, which gave her the appearance of being far older than her years. When she saw photographs of her grandmother, she decided that, if at all possible, she would do what it took to alter the inevitable. She didn't know if *anything* could be done. She was afraid that the only thing that could help would be a face-lift, and she knew she was too young for that.

The shortness of Jane's neck was compounded by excess fat under her chin and along her jawline. Nothing could be done about the former, but by removing the fat under her chin, her neckline, as well as her jawline, could be better defined.

She had the procedure done at the start of her week's vacation, allowing her to wear the chin-strap dressing almost all the time for a week. Wearing this dressing greatly reduced her postoperative swelling and allowed her to return to work on schedule.

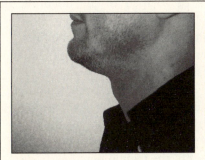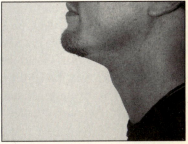

Liposuction: Before and two months postoperatively. Note the definite enhancement of the jawline.

2

Surgical Body Contouring

~

✦ Dermato Lipectomy: Panniculectomy ✦ Buttock Lifts ✦ Thigh Lifts ✦ Arm Reduction ✦ Abdominoplasty

The only thing Angela wanted for her fiftieth birthday was to be able to wear a bathing suit without a skirt.

Angela's husband, who had planned to surprise her with a birthday cruise, had to be convinced that instead, an *operation* would be a good gift. He acquiesced when Angela explained to him that it would be partially covered by their insurance plan since the surgery had been recommended by her gynecologist to relieve her chronic lower back pain. That she would look and feel better about herself was just another plus.

Angela had her operation performed in the hospital, where she spent one night. Her recuperation progressed without a problem and, by six weeks, she had regained her full energy level. She was even enrolled in an exercise class that met three times a week (see photos, page 54).

Within a year, she sent my staff a postcard from Nassau, promising to bring in the pictures of her in her new bathing suit as soon as she returned from her second honeymoon.

Long before the development of the technology that made liposuction so popular, plastic surgeons altered body contours by surgically removing excess fat and skin in almost every part of the body.

In plastic surgery, the surgical removal of skin and fat is

called *dermato lipectomy*. Incisions are made in skin folds, where they can be more easily camouflaged, reshaping pendulous bellies, drooping buttocks, and flabby thighs and arms.

Today, dermato lipectomy is usually considered secondary or ancillary to liposuction. Liposuction alone causes skin contraction, which may correct the problem entirely or will, at least, reduce the extent of any subsequent skin resection required.

While the concept of two operations instead of one may seem like double duty, in my opinion, the body is less traumatized by the two less invasive procedures than it is by a single, more extensive operation. By separating the two procedures—liposuction followed by skin resection—patients find that their recuperation time is more comfortable and, surprisingly, they are able to resume normal activity far sooner.

When Dermato Lipectomy Is the Best Choice

Even though liposuction is the current body contouring procedure of choice, dermato lipectomy still has its place, especially when there is too much skin to respond favorably to liposuction alone. The most obvious area to benefit from this type of operation is the abdomen of patients who have lost large amounts of weight (fifty pounds or more). Other areas responding to this procedure are buttocks, thighs, and arms.

The surgical procedure to resect fat and redundant skin— wherever it is on the body— may also be called *panniculectomy*, from *pannus,* the Latin word meaning *piece of cloth*.

In this chapter, we will describe how this operation is done on the abdomen. This same procedure can be tailored to buttocks, thighs, or arms. The illustration shows standard incision placements.

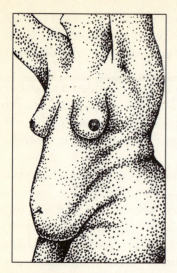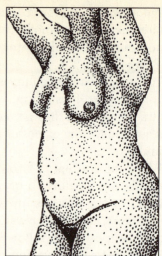

Panniculectomy (before and after), or surgical removal of an overhanging apron of fat and excess skin through a hip-to-hip incision at the pubic line, does not include diastasis recti (separated abdominal muscles). This procedure is often called for when mobility and hygiene are primary concerns.

Abdominoplasty, commonly referred to as a tummy tuck, is a more extensive related procedure coupling dermato lipectomy with repair of overly stretched abdominal muscles.

Margaret had battled her weight since her teens. Despite this, she was bright and jolly, and had worked continuously as an office manager, almost in spite of her weight, she confessed. Now in her mid-fifties, she decided that, once and for all, she didn't want to be fat anymore.

After dieting and losing seventy-five pounds, Margaret came to me for tightening. She told me that she wanted *everything* tightened but knew realistically that that wasn't possible. Since her biggest complaint was that she couldn't walk without holding her stomach out of the way, she decided to start with her belly.

Because of the amount of excess fat and skin involved, the safest and simplest procedure for Margaret was a panniculectomy, which would let her sit, stand, and walk without being encumbered by the apron of skin and fat that hung almost to her knees. She was able to walk with ease. Her recovery was dramatic, and she was able to return to work within three weeks which, because of her seniority, didn't alter her job status.

Since her operation, Margaret has lost even more weight and is now considering a face-lift.

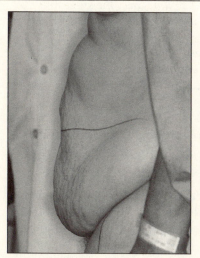 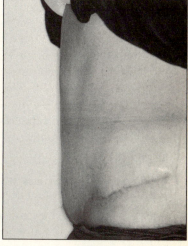

Abdominoplasty: Before, left, and three months after the operation, right. While the hip-to-hip transverse incision required for abdominoplasty will always be visible, it is easily concealed by clothing. The abdominal muscles have been tightened and liposuction has been used to contour the waist and hips. Most swelling has been resolved twelve weeks after the procedure.

Definitions Relating to Abdominal Dermato Lipectomy

Abdominoplasty (standard abdominoplasty)   A surgical procedure that removes excess fat and skin from the abdomen. Frequently, this includes tightening severely stretched abdominal muscles, from the pubis to the breastbone, and repositioning the *umbilicus*.

Dermato lipectomy   Surgical removal of excess skin and fat anywhere on the body.

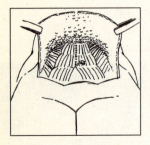

Repair of Diastasis Recti: Working through a transverse incision just above the pubic area, the surgeon repositions the navel and reconstructs the internal girdle by sewing muscles together in the midline, working from top to bottom.

Diastasis recti   The separation of the abdominus muscles, usually a result of pregnancy or massive weight gain.

Mini abdominoplasty   This is the more commonly performed procedure for less stretched muscles from the pubis to the *umbilicus*, with or without excess skin resection. It is frequently combined with liposuction. Unlike the standard abdominoplasty, the belly button is not repositioned. This procedure requires a shorter transverse incision, extending groin to groin across the pubic hairline.

Panniculectomy   A surgical procedure that removes large quantities of redundant skin and its underlying fat. Most often this operation is performed on the abdomen to remove the apron of fat and skin; however, the term can be applied to any area of the body where excess skin and fat are present, such as the upper arms. Panniculectomy is the simplest surgical solution when mobility and hygiene are primary concerns for the patient. Once this is performed, the patient might become a candidate for standard abdominoplasty, especially when additional weight is lost.

Pannus   From the Latin meaning *piece of cloth*. Used to refer to any area of excess fat and skin, most commonly the apron of fat and skin hanging from the abdomen and the flabby, winglike underarm.

Umbilicus   The navel.

Abdominal Dermato Lipectomy

Overview

In addition to removing fat and excess skin, abdominoplasty involves the tightening of separated abdominal muscles—*diastasis recti*—that may contribute to back pain and spinal problems. This condition, which does not respond to weight loss and exercise, is usually caused by repeated stretching of the muscles and skin across the abdomen through dramatic weight loss (greater than 100 pounds) or multiple or very large pregnancies.

For those with less abdominal wall damage (resulting in a potbelly deformity) a less extensive procedure, the mini abdominoplasty, may be an appropriate option.

The Procedure

Panniculectomy
The surgeon makes a transverse incision just above the pubic area, running from hipbone to hipbone. Excess skin and fat are cut away and the incision closed.

Abdominoplasty

The surgeon will make a transverse incision just above the pubic area, running from hipbone to hipbone, usually following a W pattern. A second incision is made around the navel to loosen it from surrounding tissue. After separating the skin from the abdominal wall up to the sternum and ribs, the surgeon will lift a large skin flap, exposing the abs, the vertical muscles of your abdomen. The separated muscles *(diastasis recti)* will be pulled together and sutured from pubis to sternum. This re-creates your internal girdle by tightening the abdominal wall, thus narrowing the waistline.

The skin flap is then redraped across these newly repaired muscles and the apron of excess skin and fat is removed. Then your navel will be repositioned and, if necessary, re-shaped. Finally, the incisions will be sutured and dressings applied. A temporary tube may be inserted in each side, beneath the skin, to drain excess fluid from the surgical site.

Mini Abdominoplasty

This procedure is indicated for correction of less stretched muscles and is often coupled with liposuction. It corrects the potbelly or bikini bulge deformity. Mini abdominoplasty requires a transverse incision, usually extending from groin to groin across the pubic hairline. Muscles are tightened but only from the pubis to the navel.

Length of Procedure

Panniculectomy usually takes less than one hour.

Standard abdominoplasty can take from one and a half to two and a half hours.

Mini abdominoplasty involves about one hour of surgery.

Anesthesia

Panniculectomy and standard abdominoplasty are performed under general anesthesia.

Mini abdominoplasty is usually performed under local anesthesia with sedation.

In/Outpatient

Panniculectomy and standard abdominoplasty can be performed in a hospital or your surgeon's ambulatory surgical center. Occasionally, a one-night stay is advised.

Mini abdominoplasty is usually done as an outpatient.

Pain

These are among of the most painful plastic surgery procedures; however, don't despair; this pain is easily managed with medication. Narcotic pain medication is usually prescribed for the initial recovery period. Mini abdominoplasty may require narcotic pain medication for two to three days, followed by over-the-counter medications for another week.

Incisions/Scarring

Panniculectomy: You will have a single scar across your lower abdomen, extending from hip to hip.

Standard Abdominoplasty: You will have a single scar across your lower abdomen, extending from hip to hip. You will also have a small scar around your navel as it must be moved to give your abdomen a normal appearance.

Mini Abdominoplasty: The single scar will run across the pubic hairline from groin to groin.

Scars, though permanent, usually fade over time and are placed in areas where they will be easily hidden by your underwear. You can expect it to take from nine months to a year for scars to mature. A skillful surgeon will make incisions where they are easily hidden.

Specific Risks

◆ Excessive fluid loss can lead to shock.

◆ Fluid or blood accumulation under the skin may resolve spontaneously or require surgical drainage.

◆ Skin irregularities, such as dimpling, rippling, bagginess, or asymmetry are frequent but seldom permanent. If they persist, they can usually be corrected quite easily with a second limited procedure to smooth out the skin.

◆ Dog-ear scarring, a mound of excess skin, located on the side, may require a minor skin revision performed under local anesthesia three months after the initial operation.

◆ Pigmentation changes may become permanent if the skin is exposed to the sun too soon after the operation.

◆ Blood clots in the legs (phlebitis or phlebothrombosis) are potentially serious; however, wearing compression stockings and early mobilization reduces the possibility of occurrence.

◆ Skin loss, of particular concern in patients who smoke, may result in conspicuous scarring. If this occurs, scar revision can be performed six months after the initial surgery.

Recovery Time

Return to Work
◆ Desk job:
> Panniculectomy/standard abdominoplasty: You can return to work in two to four weeks.
> Mini abdominoplasty: You can return to work after one week.
◆ Manual labor: Bending, lifting heavy weights, and straining are restricted for the first five to six weeks. Wait until your doctor gives the okay.

With a support garment, you should be increasing your activity level at a steady pace, with full return of energy and strength by six weeks. *You may take less than six weeks to get back up to speed. It's unlikely that you will take longer. These are really big operations, and you need to plan accordingly. A big mistake is not allowing yourself enough time to recuperate.*

When your surgeon uses the term *restricted activity*, pay attention. I once had a patient who had a complete tummy tuck (standard abdominoplasty). Following my instructions to arrange for someone to care for her during the first week or ten days after her operation, she dutifully arranged for her daughter to care for her during this time. While waiting for her daughter to arrive, my patient, fresh from surgery, vacuumed her house. As a result of this activity, she bled at the surgical site and developed a hematoma that required surgical drainage.

Exercise

Moderate exercise is encouraged. Start walking as soon as comfort allows. A postoperative exercise program will be recommended by your doctor to stimulate circulation and improve muscle tone. This lowers your risk of other complications.

Your doctor will monitor your progress and activity level. Strenuous exercise should be curtailed until your doctor gives the go-ahead, usually after six weeks.

Sex

Same as for exercise. Don't try anything new or strenuous for a couple of months.

Sun

Keep fresh incisions out of the sun. Always use a sunscreen.

Travel

You won't feel like taking any trips for one to two weeks following abdominoplasty. You may be up to travel after three to four days following a mini procedure.

Frequency/Duration of Results

Abdominoplasty is a procedure for women who have completed their families. Pregnancy would restretch the muscles and skin. Otherwise, results are permanent if you maintain your healthy diet and exercise regimen.

What to Expect

Expect to feel sore and constricted, and expect to need pain medication. Frequently, surgical drains are used for the first few days after abdominoplasty and sometimes after panniculectomy.

You will also be significantly limited in what you can do during the first week. Guided by your physician, you can expect a progressive return to normal activity during the second through sixth weeks.

I often recommend that patients have medical massage therapy, sometimes called lymphatic drainage massage therapy, beginning the second or third week after their operation, to relieve stiffness and promote circulation, thereby decreasing swelling. Ask your doctor if you would benefit from this treatment.

You'll be ready for your new wardrobe in about three months.

Fees/Insurance

Panniculectomy may be covered by insurance when it is indicated to facilitate mobility and promote better hygiene.

Abdominoplasty may be covered by insurance when it involves repair of muscles in the abdomen for treatment of lower back pain or spinal problems. This is one of the gray areas of plastic surgery, where cosmetic improvement is directly related to the functional repair. Ask your primary care physician to assist you in obtaining preauthorization from your insurance carrier.

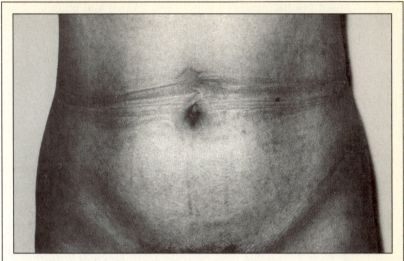

Mini-abdominoplasty: Before, above, and three months postoperatively, below. Although it is very faint, there is a short incision that extends from groin to groin across the pubic hair line. While the low rectus muscles have been tightened, the umbilicus remains in its original position. Liposuction performed at the same time added definition to the waistline.

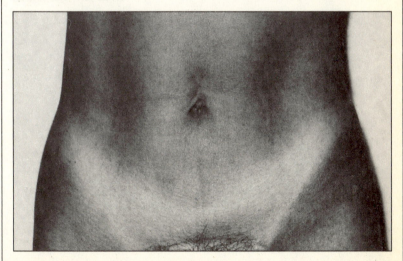

Cost for panniculectomy is between $4,000 and $5,500.

Cost for standard abdominoplasty ranges from $6,000 to $7,500.

Mini abdominoplasty costs between $3,500 and $4,500.

Important Questions to Ask About Abdominoplasty

❖ Where will the incisions be placed?

❖ Will clothing cover the scars easily? (Ask your surgeon to draw lines or dots with a marker where he plans to make incisions so you can see for yourself.)

❖ What will the skin in the treated area look like?

❖ Will there be a compression garment, and what does it look like? *(Take this into consideration when scheduling your operation, especially in hot weather.)*

❖ What is a realistic recovery timetable for me?

3

Women's Breasts

~

✦ **Augmentation Mammoplasty** ✦ **Mastopexy** ✦ **Reduction Mammoplasty** ✦ **Breast Reconstruction**

According to American Society of Plastic and Reconstructive Surgeons statistics, more than 75,000 women had *aesthetic* breast surgery during 1994. That includes breast augmentation, lifts, and reduction.

The most frequently elected surgery for women between nineteen and thirty-four, augmentation uses implants to increase a woman's bustline by one or more bra cup sizes.

Although no surgery can permanently alter the pull of gravity, a breast lift will raise and reshape sagging breasts, giving them a firmer, more attractive shape.

Breast reduction may give women with large, pendulous breasts relief from a variety of problems, from back and neck pain and irritated skin to skeletal deformities and breathing difficulties.

The best candidates for any of these breast-altering surgeries are physically healthy women who are seeking *improvement*, not *perfection*.

Definitions

Areola   The dark, pigmented area around the nipple.

Augmentation mammoplasty   Breast augmentation using implants.

Axilla   The armpit. Plural is axillae.

Breast implant   A silicone rubber shell filled with either silicone gel or inflated with a saline solution.

Capsule   Scar tissue that grows around implants or any other foreign body. Any time a foreign substance is placed in the body, the body's response is to wall it off by forming a scarlike capsule around that object.

Endoscopy   A fiber-optic technology that allows a surgeon to view images of the body's internal structures through very small incisions using a device called an *endoscope*. Some plastic surgeons use this method to position breast implants within the chest wall. Endoscopy can also assist in evaluating the condition of existing implants and the scar tissue that forms around the implant (capsule).

Gigantomastia   A medical term used to describe extremely large breasts.

Inframammary fold   The crease below the breast.

Liquid silicone   The fluid form of silicone used in the early 1960s for breast augmentation. Later disapproved for human use by the Food and Drug Administration (FDA) in 1965 because of a high complication rate.

Mammogram   Breast X ray. A diagnostic tool used not only to detect tumors but also to distinguish fat and glandular tissue.

Mammoplasty   Any operation performed on the breast.

Mastectomy   Breast removal. Usually classified as lumpectomy, simple, subtotal, total, modified radical, or radical, depending on the extent of tissue that is removed.

Mastopexy   Breast lift.

Pectoral muscles   The primary muscles of the anterior chest.

Physiologic saline   This is a saltwater solution, the same as IV saline. Closely resembling the solution that makes up approximately 71 percent of the human body, it is used to inflate saline breast implant shells to desired size.

Silicone gel   This is a jellylike form of silicone used in breast implants. Silicone gel–filled implants are no longer available except in controlled FDA studies and special cases of reconstruction.

Silicone rubber   The form of silicone used in the manufacture of the envelope or bag for breast implants.

Umbilicus   The navel.

Augmentation Mammoplasty (Breast Enlargement)

Overview

Breast augmentation or enlargement is the procedure of choice for many women who consider their breasts to be too small. This operation increases the size and alters the contour of a woman's breasts by inserting any of a variety of prostheses.

Breast augmentation is best used to enhance the breasts a full cup size, which is sufficient for most women. Anything larger may look unnatural.

Other reasons for augmentation include replacement of breast volume lost following pregnancy or simply to correct unevenness in breast size. Implants may also be used in reconstructive procedures following mastectomy.

In 97 percent of all breast augmentations, silicone rubber implants are inserted, then filled with a saline solution. Saline-filled implants should not be confused with silicone gel implants used for some twenty years but now under Food and Drug Administration review. This review was prompted by concerns regarding the health risks of silicone gel.

As of this writing, no evidence of increased cancer risk among recipients of silicone breast implants has been identified. In October 1995, the American College of Rheumatology issued a statement that "silicone implants exposed patients to no demonstrable additional risk for connective tissue or rheumatic disease." In December 1996 the American Medical Association Council on Scientific Affairs stated the position that silicone gel implants should be made available to women as long as they are made aware of all risks and benefits. At present, silicone gel–filled implants are available only to women participating in FDA-approved, manufacturer-sponsored clinical trials.

Usually, augmentation does not permanently interfere with breast sensitivity, nor does it affect fertility or pregnancy. There is a small chance, however, that it may affect your ability to nurse. Augmentation mammoplasty does not alter the effectiveness of mammography, although the mammographic technician should be made aware that you have implants.

Saline implants are more vulnerable to damage and deflation than silicone gel implants.

With both of her children in school and relatively independent, Marta was ready to return to full-time teaching. At thirty-three, she was physically active and fit, with a near-perfect figure. Her only problem was her breasts. Since having children, they had lost their volume.

Wanting to look her best when she reentered the job market, Marta asked if I could replicate the fullness she remembered when she was pregnant.

For the first couple of months, Marta wore oversized tops as she had a little difficulty becoming accustomed to the weight and fullness of her breasts. However, once she returned to her aerobics routine and started getting compliments, she began to wear more revealing clothes.

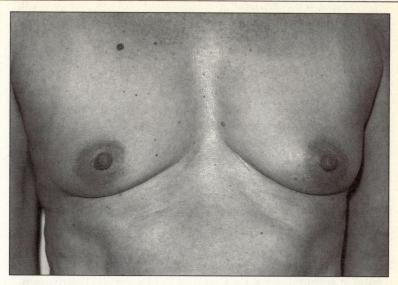

Breast Augmentation: Before, above, and two months following modest breast augmentation, below. Note, incisions are hidden in the natural fold beneath the breasts.

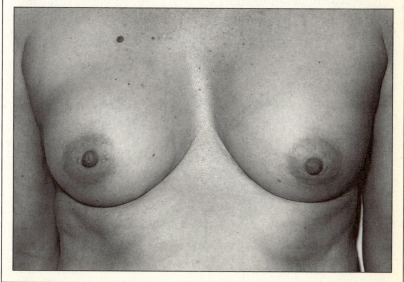

Now, ten years later, Marta is always told by her gynecologist and mammography technicians that they are
amazed at how natural her breasts look and feel.

The Procedure

This operation is designed to add fullness to the breasts by
inserting a tissue substitute—the implant—behind existing
breast tissue, either in front of or behind the pectoral muscles. A very small incision is used, relative to the size of most
implants. The incision options are: (1) around the lower half
of the areola, (2) in the inframammary fold, (3) in the axilla,
or armpits, or (4) using an endoscope, through the umbilicus (see Chapter 11, page 221).

The surgeon makes a pocket behind the breast tissue, either in front of or behind the pectoral muscle. In augmentation mammoplasty, no breast tissue is removed. The implant
is centered beneath the nipple.

The increased size of the breast mound and depth of
cleavage are determined by the size of the implant. You will
experience swelling, which may initially make you think that
you are now too big. As swelling resolves, you will feel more
comfortable with your new shape.

In this operation, there is little disruption of the mam-

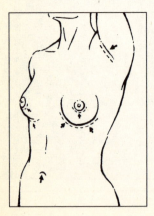

*Breast Augmentation: This procedure
requires very small incisions, relative
to the size of most implants. Incision
may be made around the lower half of
the areola; under the breasts, in the inframammary fold; in the axilla, or
armpit; or, using an endoscope,
through the umbilicus, or navel.*

mary ducts, so there is little risk of affecting the ability to breast-feed. Depending upon the degree of stretching required to accommodate the implant, temporary disruption of the sensory nerves is common, accounting for altered nipple sensation during the initial recovery period. Your sensation usually returns within three months.

Your incisions will be taped, and you will be placed in a surgical bra, which you will wear night and day, except when you shower, for one to two weeks. It is recommended to continue taping the incisions for an additional month to minimize scar widening. Expect some restriction of upper body activity during this period.

Length of Procedure

A breast augmentation operation takes one to two hours.

Anesthesia

Anesthesia is usually local with sedation.

In/Outpatient

Breast augmentation is performed in an ambulatory surgical facility or as an outpatient in a hospital.

Pain

Expect soreness requiring prescription pain medication for the first week. After that, pain can be easily managed with acetaminophen or other over-the-counter analgesics.

Incisions/Scarring

You will have incisions in one of the locations described above, positioned to be as inconspicuous as possible.

Scars will be firm and pink for six to eight weeks, and

then slowly mature and soften over several months. To minimize widening of scars, incisions are taped for six weeks after surgery. Over several months, these scars will fade. Remember that they never completely disappear.

Specific Risks

❖ Capsule formation occurs in all breast augmentations. The presence of a capsule is not a problem; however, there are three conditions of capsule formation that may require treatment: (1) the breast looks normal but it is firm to the touch; (2) the breast looks abnormal because the capsule has contracted, distorting the implant into a ball, in addition to making it feel firm to the touch; and (3) the breast looks abnormal because the capsule has contracted, and it is painful.

Usually, if you develop the first capsule condition, no treatment is recommended. For the second type—abnormal appearance—the usual protocol calls for the incision to be reopened and the capsule released. There is a chance that this contraction may recur. The third problem, contraction plus pain, usually requires repositioning the implant. If pain persists, the implants may need to be removed. Unfortunately, there is no way to predict that you will have one of these problems.

❖ Fluid or blood accumulation under the skin may resolve itself spontaneously or require surgical drainage. Excessive bleeding following the operation may cause swelling and pain. If this condition occurs, a second operation may be required to control the bleeding.

❖ Implants may break or leak. If a saline-filled implant breaks, the bag will deflate within a few hours and the salt water will be absorbed by the body.

When a gel-filled implant breaks or leaks, one of two things may occur. If the shell breaks but the capsule around it does not, there may be no detectable change in the breast. If the capsule also breaks or tears, silicone gel may move into surrounding tissue. In some cases, gel may bleed through the silicone rubber envelope into the breast, causing additional scar formation, which may be confused with a breast tumor upon physical examination. These conditions usually require an operation to remove this mass and replace the implant.

❖ Some women report that their nipples become oversensitive, undersensitive, or even numb. These are rarely permanent conditions but may persist for several months.

❖ Occasionally, implants become displaced. If this happens, the only way to get the implant back where it belongs is with another operation.

Recovery Time

Return to Work
❖ Desk job: You should be able to return to work within four to seven days.
❖ Manual labor: Bending, lifting heavy weights, and straining are restricted for three to four weeks.

Initially, using a support garment, you will increase your activity level at a steady pace, with full return of energy and strength by six weeks.

Exercise
Most patients can resume their usual level of aerobic activity two to three weeks after the operation, as long as they observe the movement restrictions noted above. Your doctor will advise you of an appropriate program.

Sex
Same as for exercise. Wait for about a week. Don't try anything new or that involves direct contact with the breasts or heavy lifting for at least three weeks.

Sun

Stay out of the sun for the first week. Always use sunscreen. Take care that incisions are not exposed to direct sun for at least six weeks.

Travel

There are no restrictions on travel by automobile, airplane, or bus. You may not feel comfortable sitting for extended periods of time for about a week.

Frequency/Duration of Results

Results are long-lasting, but the natural aging of your breasts, though slowed, is not stopped. While implants last for extended periods of time, they may need to be replaced in several years.

What to Expect

Mammography is recommended before most operations on the breast.

One of the things you will be asked to decide during your preoperative consultations is the size of the breasts you desire. A good guideline is to look for a one cup-size increase. *(Bring a nonpadded, nonunderwired bra in the cup size you think you would like with you on your first visit to assist the surgeon in sizing your implants.)*

Incisions are dressed with surgical tape. Gauze pads may be used. You may be instructed to wear a surgical bra for proper support, or your chest may be wrapped with an elastic bandage.

You must restrict your upper body movement for approximately three weeks: elbows at your sides for the first week; raising arms no more than shoulder level during the second week, and over your head during the third.

You may experience altered sensation—from numbness to

burning—in your nipples for about two weeks. This will subside as swelling resolves.

Some women experience transient increases or decreases in sensitivity of their nipples following this operation.

There may be small patches of numbness near your incisions. Usually, all numbness is resolved by three months.

If nonabsorbable sutures are used, they will be removed after a week to ten days. Swelling may take three to five weeks to subside.

You may feel more discomfort than usual during the first menstruation following your operation as your body adjusts to the implants.

Incisions may be taped for six weeks to prevent widening of the scars.

It will take a few weeks to adjust to the added weight and volume of your newly augmented breasts.

Fees/Insurance

The usual cost of breast augmentation is approximately $7,000 to $7,500 plus the cost of the implants—between $1,200 and $2,000.

This procedure is not usually covered by insurance unless it is performed as part of a medically indicated procedure such as breast reconstruction.

Important Questions to Ask About Breast Augmentation

❖ Where will the incisions be? (Ask your surgeon to draw lines or dots with a marker so you can see for yourself.)

❖ How do I decide what size I want my breasts to be?

❖ What type of implant will you use?

❖ Where will the implant be put—in front of or behind the pectoral muscles?

- What is the surgical support bra like?

- How long after my operation can I shower?

- What is a realistic recovery timetable for me?

Mastopexy (Breast Lift)

Overview

As a woman's skin loses its elasticity, her breasts often begin to sag, losing their shape and firmness. Mastopexy is a surgical procedure that raises and reshapes sagging breasts. Although no surgery can halt the sands of time, mastopexy can certainly slow them down.

Breasts of any size can be lifted, but best results are achieved in women with smaller, sagging breasts (A or B cup). Results may not last as long in heavy breasts. The ideal candidate for this procedure is a physically healthy woman who is realistic about the possible results.

Many women have mastopexy to reshape their breasts to correct stretched skin and reduced volume as a result of pregnancy and nursing. This is performed more often in recent years as an alternative to augmentation.

There is no indication that mastopexy would interfere with breast-feeding, but you may want to delay having this operation until you have completed your family, as pregnancy is liable to stretch your breasts again and offset the results of this procedure.

A breast lift won't keep your breasts firm forever. Gravity, pregnancy, aging, and weight fluctuations will eventually take their toll again. Longer-lasting results have been reported by women who have implants along with their breast lift if they want to replace lost breast mass as well as lift their breasts.

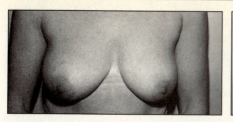
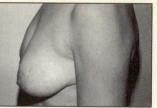

Mastopexy: Top left and right, frontal and lateral views before breast lift. Bottom left and right, six months after surgery, note that incisions are placed so that low necklines can be worn without exposing the scars.

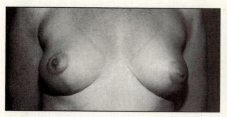
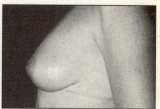

After three pregnancies—the most recent two years earlier—Rose, thirty-eight, was upset that her breasts were deflated and sagging. The nipples pointed downward.

Rose was an active runner and her loose breasts made running awkward and painful. She was forced to wear a strong support bra to keep them from flopping.

She had considered breast enlargement as a possible remedy; however, she had reservations about breast implants and opted, instead, to remove excess skin and reduce her enlarged areolas. Her nipples were raised closer to their prepregnancy position.

Since this operation only removes redundant skin, her breasts were more firm than she had imagined they would be. Rose was immediately happy to not have floppy breasts. Her biggest difficulties were the restriction on all jogging activity for the first three weeks after the operation and having to wear postoperative tape on her incisions for a full six weeks.

Once she passed these milestones, she was delighted with the look and feel of her breasts. She was also pleased that the scars were easily camouflaged.

Rose now runs without extra support.

The Procedure

Because this is primarily a skin tailoring operation, it is a relatively easy procedure for a patient to undergo. In certain circumstances, it may be done entirely under local anesthesia if there is only a small amount of correction required. In the vast majority of cases, it is done under local anesthesia with sedation.

There are several variations of incision placement. The most common uses a keyhole pattern. This allows for reduction of the diameter of the areola as well as elevation of the

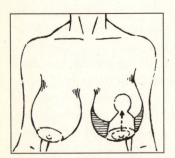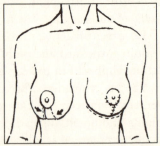

Standard incision placement for Mastopexy and Breast Reduction: Left, the arrow indicates elevation of the nipple to its new position at the top of the keyhole pattern of the incision. The shaded area indicates the segments of skin and/or breast tissue to be resected. Right, once the nipple is repositioned and the sides of the incision are closed, the resulting anchor-shaped scar is easily hidden by clothing.

nipple. Using this technique, the nipple can be raised several inches so that it is even with the inframammary crease or slightly higher. All other techniques are variations on this basic pattern. Ask your surgeon to explain the preferred approach for you.

No breast tissue is removed in mastopexy, only skin. Because of this, you will remain relatively the same size, although your breasts will seem firmer because your skin "bra" has been tightened.

In this operation, there is little disruption of the sensory nerves or the mammary ducts, so there is little risk of permanently affecting nipple sensation or the ability to subsequently breast-feed. You may be surprised that most people experience only moderate soreness rather than pain after this operation.

Your incisions will be taped, and you will be placed in a surgical bra, which you will wear night and day, except when showering, for the first week or two. It is recommended to continue taping the incisions for an additional month to minimize scar widening. Expect some restriction of upper body activity during this period.

Length of Procedure

Mastopexy takes an hour and a half to two hours.

Anesthesia

Your doctor has three choices when performing mastopexy:

Local Anesthesia: When only a small amount of correction is required, injection of anesthetic into the area being treated will be sufficient to numb it.

Local with Sedation: You will be put to sleep by medication administered through a vein. Then a local anesthetic is injected into the area being treated.

General Anesthesia: You will be put to sleep, usually using gas anesthetics, with a ventilator breathing for you.

In almost all operations, regardless of the chosen anesthetic, your doctor will also use local anesthetics with epinephrine to reduce bleeding during the operation and to aid in controlling postoperative pain.

In/Outpatient

Breast lift surgery is usually done in a walk-in surgical facility or in the hospital on an outpatient basis.

Pain

Postoperative pain can be easily relieved with medication prescribed by your physician for the first few days, then by over-the-counter pain medication.

Incisions/Scarring

Mastopexy scars are permanent; however, they are generally positioned so that you can wear strapless tops and low necklines.

Specific Risks

- ◆ Skin loss due to inadequate blood flow is a frequent problem for smokers and may result in significant scars that require subsequent revision.

- ◆ Fluid or blood accumulation under the skin usually resolves itself spontaneously.

- ◆ Asymmetry often reflects the preoperative condition of the breast. If there is a big discrepancy in the size of your breasts, you may wish to even them out at this time.

✦ Scar pigmentation changes may become permanent if the skin is exposed to the sun soon after the operation.

✦ Temporary change in nipple sensation is common, but permanent sensory changes are unlikely.

Recovery Time

Return to Work
✦ Desk job: You should feel like returning to work after three to four days.
✦ Manual labor: Bending, lifting heavy weights, and straining are restricted for three weeks.

With a support or surgical bra, you should be increasing your activity level at a steady pace, with full return of energy and strength by six weeks.

Exercise
Most patients can resume their usual level of aerobic activity a week after the operation, although contact sports are not advised. You *must* wear a support bra when you first resume exercise.

You can expect to resume weight training after three to four weeks with your physician's go-ahead.

Sex
Same as for exercise. Wait for about a week. Don't try anything that puts pressure on the breasts for four to six weeks.

Sun
Stay out of the sun for the first week. Always use sunscreen.

Travel
There are no restrictions on travel by automobile, airplane, or bus. You may not feel comfortable sitting for extended periods of time for about a week.

Frequency/Duration of Results

With time, the ratio of fat to breast tissue increases. This has little to do with *being* fat, but rather is a reflection of the natural aging process. The more fat content in your breasts, the more your breasts will sag and the less firm they will be.

What to Expect

Breasts will be bruised, swollen, and achy for two to three days following the operation. You will wear an elastic bandage or surgical bra over gauze dressings for three or four days. This will be replaced by a soft support bra that must be worn day and night for up to four weeks.

Nonabsorbable sutures will be removed after a week. Incisions are often taped for six weeks to reduce widening of scars.

Breast skin may be very dry following surgery and should be moisturized several times a day. Do not tug at your skin and do not apply this lotion to the sutured areas.

Postoperative swelling may cause some loss of feeling in the nipples and numbness in the breast tissues. This will subside over the next six to eight weeks.

Fees/Insurance

The usual cost of mastopexy is between $3,500 and $5,000.

This procedure is not usually covered by insurance unless it is performed as part of a medically indicated procedure.

Important Questions to Ask About Breast Lifts

❖ Which surgical approach is recommended, and why?

❖ Where will the scars be located? (Ask your surgeon to draw them with a marker to show where incisions will be made.)

✦ Will I have to wear a special bra? For how long?

✦ What is a realistic recovery timetable for me?

✦ How long after my operation before I can take a shower?

✦ What restrictions are there on movement and activities?

Reduction Mammoplasty (Breast Reduction)

Overview

The goal of this procedure is to give a woman with cumbersome breasts relief from a variety of medical problems caused by the weight and size of her breasts. Bra straps, even wide ones, may groove the shoulders, while underwire bras poke and irritate skin under and at the sides of the breasts. Extremely heavy breasts have been charged with a variety of medical problems such as back and neck pain, skeletal deformities, and breathing difficulties.

Breast reduction surgery is also especially beneficial to the woman or teenage girl who is painfully self-conscious of her breast size.

Whenever a patient tells me that her spouse doesn't understand why she wants breast reduction, I suggest that she divide five pounds of potatoes into two bags, tie the handles together with a length of string, and then have her partner wear this pendant around his neck for a couple of hours. That usually stops all future "But honey, I love you the way you are" conversations.

In breast reduction, your plastic surgeon not only operates to reduce the size of your breasts but also is called upon to be a sculptor to shape them.

At sixteen, Zena already had DD breasts. Her mother, a dressmaker, made most of her clothes so that her disproportionately large breasts were camouflaged, but

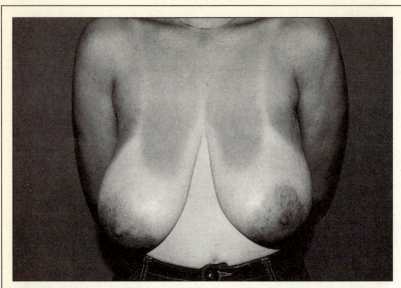

Breast reduction: Before, above, and four months postoperatively, below. The boxy or square appearance can be expected to resolve within a year.

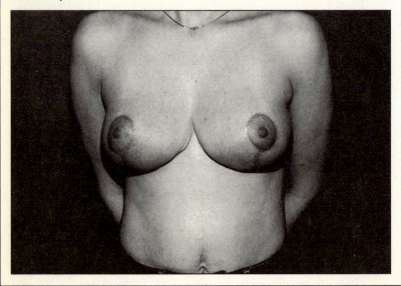

Zena did not participate in phys. ed.; did not shower with the other girls, and would not go to the beach.

Zena's father, an Eastern European immigrant, initially opposed this operation, fearing that it would affect his daughter's marriageability, but he yielded to his wife's intervention on Zena's behalf.

Zena was realistic in her expectations. She did not want *small* breasts. She decided that a full B or small C cup would still be full on her frame but would be considerably more manageable. Over a school break, she had the procedure done in a hospital and, because her mother was taking care of her, went straight home. By the time classes resumed, she was comfortable enough to return to school, although she didn't carry her heavy book bag for several weeks.

About five pounds of breast tissue were removed in this operation. Because of the nature of Zena's skin, her scars were thicker than ideal, but the relief of the weight and size of her breasts more than compensated for this. She declined scar revision because she did not want to interfere with her school activities.

The Procedure

Breast reduction is almost always done under general anesthesia in a hospital. If large amounts of breast resection and associated blood loss are anticipated, you may be asked to donate a unit of your own blood one or two weeks prior to the operation so it may be given back to you during or after your operation.

The standard incision follows the keyhole pattern, described in the mastopexy section (see page 78). All other approaches are variations of this technique. In extreme cases of gigantomastia, a free-nipple graft technique may be necessitated due to the distance that the nipple must be raised.

In this variation, the nipple and areola are transferred as a skin graft to their new position.

In most operations, the areola is reduced first, then the excess skin is resected, creating a pedicle or tissue base that is used to carry the nipple to its new location at the top of the keyhole. This allows for several inches of nipple translocation. Excess breast tissue is removed from the top and sides of the pedicle to create the desired size and shape. The dissection extends down to the muscles of the chest wall. The depth of this dissection explains why muscles feel so sore after breast reduction surgery.

A drain is placed on each side to evacuate any old blood and prevent fluid accumulation. These are usually left in place until the draining stops, usually after three to seven days.

The incisions are sutured and taped. You will be placed in a surgical bra padded with gauze. Sometimes a one-night hospital stay is suggested, but most people go home the same day.

Expect to be sore and require narcotic prescription pain medication for up to one week. Sponge baths are mandatory until the drains are removed. You will continue to wear the support bra night and day except when showering for the first two to three weeks. It is recommended that you tape incisions for an additional month to minimize scar widening. Upper body activity is restricted until your doctor approves increased motion.

Your surgeon may recommend that you take an iron supplement (not merely a multivitamin with iron) before surgery and for three months afterward to build up the iron in your body. This will help replenish any blood lost during the operation and will help you to regain your preoperative energy levels at a faster pace.

Length of Procedure

Breast reduction takes two to three hours.

Anesthesia

The majority of breast reduction operations are done under general anesthesia.

In/Outpatient

Breast reduction surgery can be done as an outpatient procedure, but a one-night hospital stay may be recommended in individual cases.

Pain

You will feel pain for the first two to three days, especially when you move or cough. You may be given breathing exercises to do to keep your lungs clear. Use your prescription pain medication as needed for comfort.

You will be sore for a week or longer at which point any residual discomfort is easily controlled with over-the-counter medications.

Incisions/Scarring

Scars, though permanent, fade over time. They are generally positioned so that they can be hidden easily by clothing.

Scars should be taped for the first six weeks after surgery to prevent widening.

Specific Risks

- ❖ Excessive fluid loss can lead to shock.

- ❖ Fluid or blood accumulation under the skin may resolve itself spontaneously or require surgical drainage.

- ❖ Scars may widen or thicken, requiring revision at a later time.

❖ Pigmentation changes may become permanent if scars are exposed to the sun soon after the operation.

❖ Lost of skin or loss of a part or all of the nipple is of greater concern for patients who smoke.

Recovery Time

Return to Work
❖ Desk job: You should feel like returning to work after two to three weeks.
❖ Manual labor: Bending, lifting heavy weights, and straining are restricted for four to six weeks.

With the support of a surgical bra, you should be increasing your activity level at a steady pace, with full return of energy and strength by six weeks. Some patients who have a smaller reduction require less time; few take longer.

Exercise
Most patients slowly resume aerobic activity. Start walking as soon as comfort allows. Your surgeon will assist you in formulating a suitable, graduated exercise regimen.

Sex
Let comfort dictate. Wait for about a week. Avoid doing anything that involves direct contact with the breasts or heavy lifting for two weeks.

Sun
Stay out of the sun for the first week. Always use sunscreen.

Travel
There are no restrictions on travel by automobile, airplane, or bus. You may not feel comfortable with extended travel for two weeks.

Frequency/Duration of Results

Results are permanent. However, if this procedure is done during the teen years, there is a small chance of continued breast growth. In adult women, this is not likely.

What to Expect

A mammogram is often suggested before any operation on the breast.

After your operation, you will be wrapped in an elastic bandage or placed in a surgical bra over gauze dressings.

A small tube may be placed in each breast to drain off blood and fluids. You may be asked to empty the drain reservoir if necessary. *Make sure that you are instructed in drain management before your operation, preferably in your doctor's office.*

You also may be given breathing exercises to perform after your operation. *Make sure you are instructed in how to do them properly during your preoperative consultation with the anesthesiologist or respiratory therapist.*

Bandages will be removed a day or two after the operation. You will wear a surgical bra at all times (except when bathing) for three to four weeks, until swelling and bruising subside.

Postoperative swelling may cause loss of feeling in the nipples and numbness of the breast skin. This usually subsides over the next three months.

Sutures will be removed in one to two weeks.

Incisions will often be taped for six weeks to prevent widening of the scars.

In large reductions, expect that your breasts will look square rather than rounded. As you heal, the natural weight of the breast will round out the contour.

Fees/Insurance

The usual cost of reduction mammoplasty is $5,500 to $7,000.

This procedure is usually covered by insurance when performed as part of a medically indicated procedure to treat neck, back, and shoulder pain or other problems relating to the spine. These complaints should be verified in writing by your primary care physician preoperatively.

Important Questions to Ask About Breast Reduction

- How many scars will there be?

- Where will the scars be located? (Ask your surgeon to draw lines or dots with a marker where incisions will be made so you can see for yourself.)

- What operative approach will be needed?

- Will I require a blood transfusion?

- May I donate my own blood in advance of my operation in case I do need a transfusion?

- What is the surgical bra like?

- Should I take any special vitamin and iron supplements before and after my operation? If so, for how long after?

- What is a realistic recovery timetable for me?

Breast Reconstruction

Mildred is a fifty-three-year-old manager of a dental office who had her left breast removed for cancer two years before coming to me for reconstruction. She required no additional cancer therapy and has no residual sign of disease. Her remaining breast was a D cup.

Her primary complaint was difficulty in dressing. She wore a prosthesis, but found it difficult to manage. Her request was that I give her a breast mound so that she could have symmetry. If possible, she also wanted her remaining breast reduced. She had no desire to have nipple reconstruction done, and she did not want extensive flap operations performed.

For the first stage, she had a tissue expander placed in her chest. Over the course of three months, this device was inflated with saline solution to a size larger than she ultimately wanted to have. As a second stage, the expander was replaced with a smaller permanent prosthesis, which formed the new breast mound and fold.

Mildred's other breast was then reduced to a large B cup size, proportionate to the reconstructed side.

Not only was she pleased that she had her breast mound back, she was delighted that dressing was no longer a chore.

Overview

Fortunately, treatment of cancer of the breast no longer requires extensive mutilating operations. This is a result of earlier detection and advances in adjuvant therapies.

There is also a new awareness among cancer surgeons who recognize the necessity of treating the *whole* patient, not just her cancerous breast. Many women will not be grateful that a mastectomy was performed to save their lives when they have been left deformed.

Removal of even a portion of a woman's breast can lead to a request for reconstruction. This may take the form of comparable reduction of the other breast or replacing missing volume with a small breast implant.

When an entire breast has been removed, options of reconstruction include placement of an implant alone, transpositioning of muscle and skin—with or without an implant—or microsurgical transfer of skin and muscle. Each of these procedures has advantages and unique risks. Timing of reconstruction ranges from immediate (at the time of your cancer operation) to delayed. The selection of reconstructive method will depend upon not only your medical condition but also the amount and condition of your remaining chest wall tissue and any need for adjuvant cancer treatments.

The first person you will consult to discuss reconstruction will most likely be your cancer surgeon, not a plastic surgeon. It is appropriate to discuss your reconstruction options *before* any cancer operation is performed. If this is not a comfortable thing for you to do, or if you have already had a mastectomy, there is no time limit on discussing your options for reconstruction *afterward*.

4

The Eyelids

~

◆ **Upper Blepharoplasty**
◆ **Lower Blepharoplasty** ◆ **Blepharoplasty for Asians**

The eyes, commonly referred to as the windows of the soul, say a great deal about a person. We evaluate people's moods or attitudes by the light in their eyes or its absence. We decide whether or not people have integrity by how they look us in the eye.

Not surprisingly, when what a person projects doesn't match what he or she feels, that person often turns to plastic surgery. I've heard people say, "I must really look horrible today. Everyone keeps asking me if I'm sick. It's odd; I'm feeling great."

When patients tell me that they always *look* tired, or that they can't understand why they look like they haven't slept in a week, I suggest that we take a close look at their eyelids. Likewise, when a patient is considering improving multiple areas but doesn't know where to start, the eyelids are a very good place to begin. Contrary to the perception that you have to be of a certain age before you need to have your eyes done, young adults may also benefit from removing bags under the eyes or lifting heavy lids.

Overview

Operations on the eyelids are not only among the most commonly performed plastic surgery procedures but also the ones that give a high degree of improvement and satisfaction for a minimal investment of time and money.

If you have the opportunity to speak with anyone who has had an eyelid procedure, they will more than likely tell you that it was as close to painless as they could imagine. Another attraction is the relative ease of recovery. Frequently, tinted glasses are all that is needed to be able to resume most daily activity, including work.

For these reasons, blepharoplasty is commonly the first operation many cosmetic surgery patients undertake.

Definitions

Blepharoplasty   A term generally used to describe cosmetic surgical procedures performed on the eyelids.

Cilia   Eyelashes.

Conjunctiva   The inner lining of the eyelids.

Cornea   The clear, sensitive covering of the eyeball.

Corneal abrasion   A scratch of the cornea that causes intense pain and may result in visual impairment if not treated appropriately.

Corneal ulceration   A painful, crater-shaped interruption of the corneal surface caused by dry eye, which may lead to infection, scarring, and visual impairment if not treated appropriately.

Dry eye   Inadequate lubrication of the eyeball due to *lagophthalmos*—inability to fully close the eye—or insufficient tear production, which can lead to corneal ulceration.

Ectropion   A term used to describe the abnormal eversion of the lower eyelid, a condition also called *bloodhound eyes*.

Entropion   A term used to describe the abnormal inversion, or inward turn, of the lower eyelid, causing the lashes to rub against and irritate the eyeball.

Lagophthalmos   Inability to fully close the upper eyelid. When caused by postoperative swelling, it is self-limited. A rare but more serious problem is lagophthalmos due to contracture, or shortening, of the upper eyelid muscles or skin. This condition may require surgical correction.

Laser blepharoplasty   Standard blepharoplasty supplemented with the use of the laser.

Milia   Cysts that look like whiteheads, which may form along suture lines. Treatment requires unroofing or shaving off the top of the cyst so that it may heal from the bottom up.

Palpebral Fold   The crease in the upper eyelid. It is used as an approach for resection of excess skin and fat from the upper lid. Its position characterizes an eye as being Oriental or Occidental.

Ptosis   Drooping of the upper eyelid, usually caused by weakness or detachment of the levator muscle, which raises the upper lid.

Sclera   The white part of the eyeball.

Scleral hematoma   A black-and-blue mark on the sclera, which appears as a cherry red spot. It resolves over a two- to three-week period.

Scleral show   A result of ectropion, caused by the retraction of the lower eyelid, which exposes the sclera below the pupil of the eye when looking straight ahead.

Subciliary incision   A lower blepharoplasty incision placed on the outside of the lower eyelid, just below the eyelashes.

Transconjunctival incision   A lower blepharoplasty incision placed on the inside of the lower eyelid.

Upper Blepharoplasty

A common eyelid problem that betrays age is drooping upper lids. While heavily hooded eyes may be viewed as sexy or sultry on the movie screen, more often they make you look old and tired. In addition, such redundant skin may also impair vision.

Carlos was a fifty-one-year-old hardware store owner with three daughters, the youngest of whom was "finally

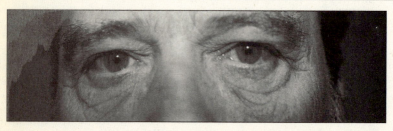

Upper and Lower Blepharoplasty: Before, top, and three weeks after, bottom, the procedure. Excess fat and skin were removed from both the upper and lower eyelids. There is still some redness around the eyes. As soon as the swelling subsided, the patient commented that his peripheral vision was improved.

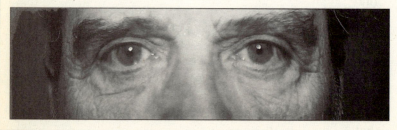

getting married" in four months. Despite the family's joy as wedding plans were made, Carlos was secretly stinging over something his future son-in-law's aunt had said at the engagement party more than a year earlier: "Oh, I thought you were the grandfather."

His wife had told him not to let it bother him, but Carlos wanted to look his best. Nobody was going to accuse him of being an *old* man.

Carlos not only had problems with bags and too much skin under his eyes, but also drooping upper eyelids. This latter condition also impaired his peripheral vision, somewhat like blinders on a horse. This had developed so gradually that Carlos was not aware that he had a problem until his field of vision was checked during his preoperative examination.

In one operation, he had the excess skin and fat removed on the upper eyelids, using an incision that followed the natural skin crease of the lid. Similarly, through an incision just below the lower eyelashes, excess skin was resected from the lower lids and the bulging fat removed. As soon as the swelling had subsided, Carlos commented that his side vision was markedly improved. He noticed this, especially, when he was able to parallel park his car on the first try.

When the wedding day came, no one could mistake Carlos for anything *but* the proud *father* of the bride.

The Procedure

The goal of upper eyelid blepharoplasty is to rejuvenate the face by restoring the shape of the eye. Removing redundant skin and fat simultaneously corrects any vision impairment resulting from this hooding.

Upper blepharoplasty is usually performed under local anesthesia with sedation. The surgeon draws an incision that follows the palpebral (upper eyelid) fold and extends slightly to the outside of the eye socket. A second line is drawn to include all of the redundant skin. This strip of skin is then excised and the individual pockets of fat that lie below are entered and the excess is removed. This does not require any contact with the eyeball itself.

The incision is closed, frequently with dissolving sutures, and then taped with surgical strips. A protective ointment is placed on the eyeball for lubrication. During the first twenty-four hours, cold compresses are applied to the lids to reduce swelling and bruising.

Length of Procedure

Upper eyelid blepharoplasty takes between forty-five minutes and an hour.

Anesthesia

Local anesthesia with sedation is commonly used in this procedure.

In/Outpatient

Upper eyelid blepharoplasty is generally performed in an ambulatory surgery facility as an outpatient.

Pain

This truly is as close to pain-free plastic surgery as you can get. You may be given prescription pain medication, but it is unlikely that you will need to use it for more than a day, if at all.

CAUTION: Pain may be a sign of a problem. Should you experience pain that does not readily respond to your medication, contact your doctor immediately.

Incisions/Scarring

The incisions follow the palpebral fold of your upper eyelids.
Initially, the incisions will be red but, within three to six
months, they tend to heal so well that they are often described
as "disappearing." *Anyone—men included—may wish to stop
at the makeup counter and pick up some camouflage tricks.*

Specific Risks

❖ Lagophthalmos (sleeping with your eyes open) may occur
immediately after an operation but resolves in a matter of
days. If it persists, artificial tears or ophthalmic ointment
may be prescribed to prevent corneal injury. This condition usually corrects itself and rarely requires a secondary
corrective procedure.

❖ Dry eye syndrome may develop secondary to lagophthalmos
or can occur in patients who have borderline or decreased
tear production. This condition requires frequent use of artificial tears or ophthalmic ointment to prevent corneal injury. *Advise your surgeon before this operation if you use or
require eyedrops of **any** type on a daily basis. This includes the
over-the-counter products that take away redness.*

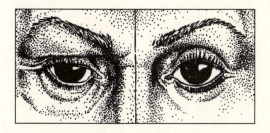

*Upper and Lower Blepharoplasty: Incisions for upper and
lower eyelid lifts appear as lines which could be creases so
that they are not noticeable.*

❖ Milia may occur along the external incision line and requires unroofing, or shaving off the top of the cyst, so that it heals itself.

❖ You have no risk of blindness if you have blepharoplasty. This is an eye*lid* procedure, not an eye*ball* procedure.

❖ Scar pigmentation may become permanent if the scar is exposed to the sun soon after the operation.

Recovery Time

Return to Work
❖ Desk job: You will be allowed to return to work in three or four days; most people wait a full week to allow for resolution of bruising.
❖ Manual labor: Bending, lifting heavy weights, or straining are restricted. Consult your surgeon before resuming any heavy work.

Exercise
Most patients can resume their usual level of aerobic activity a week after the operation.

Once bruising has disappeared, feel free to resume weight training as well. Your doctor can help you develop an appropriate schedule.

Sex
Same as for heavy exercise.

Sun
Stay out of the sun. Always use sunscreen and wear sunglasses.

Travel
There are no restrictions on travel by automobile, airplane, or bus.

Frequency/Duration of Results

Results are permanent. This is usually a one-time operation.

What to Expect

Expect two black eyes. You may or may not get them. If you do, it takes a week to ten days for them to resolve. A scleral hematoma, while less common, requires two to three weeks to resolve.

Expect to look worse before you look better. Prepare family—and especially small children—for this prior to having your operation.

You will look worse than you feel. Let those close to you know that this is part of the recovery process.

The lubricating ointment placed in your eye after your operation will cause initial blurring of vision, which may last for one to two days. *Don't plan on driving or doing close work, such as reading, watching TV, or working at your computer during this time.*

You will need to keep your head elevated at all times, even while sleeping, for the first week, as this will reduce bruising and swelling. *A recliner will keep you in the proper position.*

Cold compresses are generally applied at frequent intervals for the first twenty-four hours to minimize bruising and swelling. *Frozen peas in a zip-top plastic bag wrapped in a hand towel make an excellent compress.*

After twenty-four hours, you may find that warm compresses help to resolve bruising and swelling. *Some patients prefer to continue cold compresses during this time; most find warm compresses beneficial.*

Surgical tape and/or sutures are removed within a week after your operation.

Following tape and/or suture removal, your incisions will appear as red lines for the first few weeks and may be camouflaged by tinted glasses. *If you wear glasses, your op-*

tometrist can put a temporary tint in them so you won't have to buy new lenses. Green, brown, and gray tones work best. The tint can be removed later, if you desire. If you don't wear glasses, get a pair of nonprescription lenses with a suitable tint. Dark sunglasses are hard to wear indoors.

Your eyelids will not function normally for the first week or two due to swelling. *To avoid eyestrain, give your eyes a break every two hours or so by covering them with a warm towel for a few minutes. Don't wait until your eyes feel tired. Set a clock and follow a schedule.*

Your eyes will not look normal to you for the first few weeks while swelling is resolving. Don't be alarmed if you think you look strange during this time. Asymmetry—one eye looking differently—is common, and usually reflects your preoperative condition. *Study your eyes beforehand, and you will see that they are not perfectly matched. Seek balance, not perfect symmetry.*

Because your eyelids are not working optimally, you will not be allowed to wear contact lenses for about two weeks after your operation. *Wearing glasses rather than contacts actually works to your advantage as glasses tend to camouflage your bruising.*

Some patients who wear glasses may find that they need to change their prescription after undergoing blepharoplasty. This is not because of a change in the eyeball but because they are opening their lids wider.

Fees/Insurance

The usual cost of upper blepharoplasty is between $3,500 and $5,000. Cost of having upper and lower blepharoplasty is between $5,000 and $6,500.

This procedure is not usually covered by insurance unless it is performed to correct significant visual field impairment. You may be required to obtain a visual field examination to document your impairment. Consult your insurance carrier and primary care physician to determine if you qualify for reimbursement.

Important Questions to Ask About Upper Eyelid Blepharoplasty

❖ Where will the scars be?

❖ Will I have sutures that will need to be removed?

❖ When will I be able to wear my contact lenses again?

❖ When may I apply makeup again?

❖ What is a realistic recovery timetable for me?

Lower Blepharoplasty

Bags under the eyes plague old and young alike. They also account for the dark ring under the eye, which is most obvious in overhead light. Many patients think this is a skin pigmentation problem, when it is, in most cases, a shadow.

Lower eyelid plasty may be combined with an upper eyelid procedure or, more commonly in the younger person, performed alone.

Gail was a twenty-eight-year-old account executive for an advertising agency. In order to maintain the stamina required for her to stay on the fast track required by her job, Gail was conscientious about staying healthy, eating sensibly, exercising regularly, and getting sufficient rest. Despite all of this attention to well-being, she bore the brunt of early-morning comments from her coworkers, who accused her of leading a wild, single lifestyle. Even after a full night's sleep, she would be asked if she was tired or ill or if something had happened to make her sad.

When Gail came to the office with the complaint that she always looked worse than she felt, it was obvious that the source of her problem was the puffiness or bags under her eyes. On further questioning, she said that she looked just like her father and was really worried that she was going to end up looking like her grandmother who had *huge* bags under her eyes.

Her problem was excess fat under the eye, which had nothing to do with obesity. Anatomically, the eyeball is surrounded by a cushion of fat held in place by a membrane which, in some people, weakens. This allows the fat to bulge and form what we call bags. This weakness can be acquired over time or, as in Gail's case, may be genetically determined.

Gail wanted to know if it was too early for her to start having cosmetic plastic surgery done. I explained to her that, while it might be beneficial to wait to have some

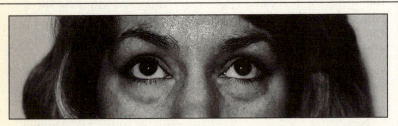

Lower Blepharoplasty: Before, above, and six months postoperative, below. Incisions for the procedure were placed on the inside of the lower eyelids.

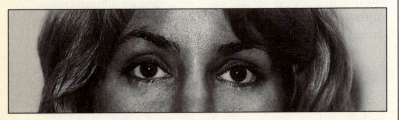

procedures, there would be no health or cosmetic reason to postpone correcting her condition. Usually, lower eyelid operations of this type are performed only once. Aging might produce loose, wrinkled skin but not more fat.

Because her only problem was excess fat, not excess or loose skin from aging—one of the benefits of doing the procedure early—Gail was given the option of having the incision placed on the inside of the lower eyelid (the transjunctival approach). This allowed her to return to work, looking totally rested, after a week's "vacation." Not only did the comments stop, but her responsibilities were increased . . . perhaps because she always looks like she is up to anything her boss throws her way.

The Procedure

Lower blepharoplasty is usually performed under local anesthesia with sedation. There are two surgical approaches to the lower eyelid. The most common technique utilizes a subciliary incision, which allows for removal of the excess fat. This approach also allows for removal of any redundant skin.

The second approach utilizes the transconjunctival incision through which excess fat alone is removed. This is most useful in the patient who has no need for skin resection or the patient who does not want to deal with an external scar.

Neither incision requires any contact with the eyeball itself.

The external incision is closed, frequently with dissolving sutures. The lids are taped with surgical strips. A lubricating ointment is frequently placed on the eyeball. Cold compresses are applied to reduce swelling and bruising.

Length of Procedure

Lower blepharoplasty takes between forty-five minutes and an hour.

Anesthesia

Local anesthesia with sedation is the most common method used in this procedure.

In/Outpatient

Lower blepharoplasty is generally performed in an ambulatory surgery facility as an outpatient.

Pain

This truly is as close to pain-free plastic surgery as you can get. You may be given prescription pain medication, but it is unlikely that you will need to use it for more than a day, if at all. *Pain may be indicative of a problem. Should you experience pain that does not readily respond to your medication, contact your doctor immediately.*

Incisions/Scarring

The subcilliary incision is placed just below your lower lash line. Initially, the incisions will be red, but within three to six months, they tend to heal so well that often they are described as disappearing.

The transjunctival incision is placed inside the lower lid. There is no external scar.

Specific Risks

* Scleral show, initially, may be caused by swelling. Treatment involves extended surgical taping of the lower eyelids until the swelling resolves. There is usually no need for secondary operative intervention. In the rare case when this does not respond, a corrective operation is performed to reposition the lower lid.

❖ Milia may occur along an external incision line. Treatment requires unroofing, or shaving off the top of the cyst, so that it heals itself.

❖ You have no risk of blindness if you have blepharoplasty. This is an eye*lid* procedure, not an eye*ball* procedure.

❖ Scar pigmentation may become permanent if the skin is exposed to the sun soon after the operation.

Recovery Time

Return to Work
❖ Desk job: You will be allowed to return to work in three or four days; most people wait a full week to allow bruising to resolve.
❖ Manual labor: Bending, lifting heavy weights, or straining are restricted for one week.

Exercise
Most patients can resume their usual level of aerobic activity a week after the operation.
Once bruising has disappeared, feel free to resume weight training as well.

Sex
Same as for exercise. Wait for about a week. Don't try anything new or strenuous for a couple of weeks.

Sun
Stay out of the sun for the first week. Always use sunscreen and wear sunglasses.

Travel
There are no restrictions on travel by automobile, airplane, or bus.

Frequency/Duration of Results

Results are permanent. This is usually a one-time operation.

What to Expect

Expect two black eyes, but you may or may not get them. If you do, it takes a week to ten days for them to resolve. A scleral hematoma may require two to three weeks to resolve.

Expect to look worse before you look better. Prepare family—and especially small children—for this prior to having your operation.

You will look worse than you feel. Let those close to you know that this is part of the recovery process.

The lubricating ointment placed in your eye after your operation will cause initial blurring of vision, which may last for one to two days. *Don't plan on driving or doing close work, such as reading, watching TV, and working at your computer during this time.*

You will need to keep your head elevated at all times, including at night, for the first week as this will reduce bruising and swelling. *A recliner will keep you in the proper position.*

Cold compresses are generally applied at frequent intervals for the first twenty-four hours to minimize bruising and swelling. *Frozen peas in a zip-top plastic bag wrapped in a hand towel make an excellent compress.*

After twenty-four hours, you may find that warm compresses help to resolve bruising and swelling. *Some patients prefer to continue cold compresses during this time; most find warm compresses beneficial.*

Surgical tape and/or sutures are removed within a week after your operation.

Following tape and/or suture removal, an external incision will appear as a red line for the first few weeks and may be camouflaged by tinted glasses. *If you wear glasses, your optometrist can put a temporary tint in them so you won't have to buy new lenses. This tint can be removed later if you desire. If you don't wear glasses, get a pair of nonprescription lenses with a tint. Dark sunglasses are hard to wear indoors.*

Your eyelids may not function normally for the first week or two due to swelling. *To avoid eyestrain, give your eyes a break every two hours or so by covering them with a warm towel for a few minutes. Don't wait until your eyes feel tired. Set a clock and follow a schedule.*

Your eyes will not look normal to you for the first few weeks while swelling is resolving. Don't be alarmed if you think you look strange during this time. Asymmetry—one eye looking differently—is common, and usually reflects your preoperative condition. *Study your eyes beforehand and you will see that they are not perfectly matched. Seek balance, not perfect symmetry.*

Because your eyelids are not working optimally, you will not be allowed to wear contact lenses for about two weeks after your operation. *Wearing glasses rather than contacts actually works to your advantage as glasses tend to camouflage your bruising.*

A man who requires a subcilliary incision might consider paying a visit to the cosmetic counter for some tips on how to use a concealer to mask any discoloration.

When a transjunctival approach is used, expect some degree of intermittent drainage from your eyes. Most obvious upon waking in the morning, this is potentially disturbing if not anticipated. It will decrease over seven to ten days. *Place an old towel on your pillow to prevent stains.*

Fees/Insurance

The usual cost of lower blepharoplasty is between $3,500 and $5,000. Cost of having upper and lower blepharoplasty is between $5,000 and $6,500.

This procedure is not usually covered by insurance.

Important Questions to Ask About
Lower Eyelid Blepharoplasty

❖ Where will the scars be?

❖ Will I have sutures that will need to be removed?

❖ When will I be able to wear my contact lenses again?

❖ When may I apply makeup again?

❖ What is a realistic recovery timetable for me?

Blepharoplasty for Asians

The most common cosmetic procedure requested by Asians is blepharoplasty to give their faces a more Western, or Occidental, appearance. This is achieved by creating an upper eyelid fold.

If you are such a patient, be sure that you seek out a plastic surgeon who is experienced in this procedure and who understands your wishes. Often Occidental blepharoplasty is combined with cosmetic rhinoplasty to augment and elevate the bridge of the nose, also contributing to a more Western appearance.

5

The Nose

~

❖ Rhinoplasty ❖ Septoplasty

The nose is one of the most dominant and distinctive features of the human body. Its central location only serves to confirm its importance. However, when it is the center of attention as well, you can be relatively certain that something is out of balance.

Not surprisingly, rhinoplasty is among the oldest of plastic surgery operations. To this day, it remains among the most frequently requested cosmetic procedure by both men and women, young and old. Reasons for such requests range from removing a prominent hump or straightening a crook to opening an airway.

Overview

There are two main reasons for operating on the nose. The results of one is seen; the other, unseen.

The more obvious of the two is rhinoplasty, or the nose job. This is a procedure that shapes and alters the appearance of the external nose. It may require rasping or moving the nasal bones, carving or resecting portions of nasal cartilage, and redraping the nasal skin.

At sixteen, Dawn was your typical mortified teen. She had spent her freshman, sophomore, and junior years in high school facing the cruel wisecracks from classmates about her prominent nose. She spent many a tearful night staring into a mirror, wishing for something other than her father's nose.

This prompted her to launch an all-out campaign for a nose job. That was all she wanted for her high school

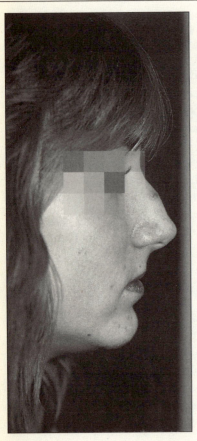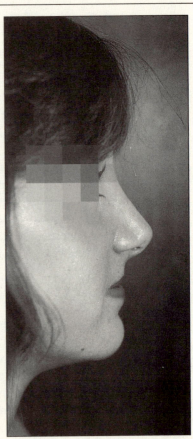

Rhinoplasty: Before, left, and four months after, right. The procedure involved reduction and refinement of the prominent basal bones and the nasal tip cartilage.

graduation present . . . and she wanted it before her senior year. Her parents acquiesced and, during the summer after her junior year, she came to me to have her
nose, as she put it, "fixed." Her goal was simply to improve her profile and make her nose smaller. This required reduction and refinement of both the prominent
nasal bones and the nasal tip cartilage.

Dawn happily returned to school for her senior year,
delighted that her yearbook picture would document her
new image. Even her younger brother conceded that she
looked okay.

Results of septoplasty are usually considered functional
rather than cosmetic. In this procedure, a deviation of the
septum is straightened, opening the airways, thereby making breathing easier. A septoplasty can be performed with no
obvious alteration in the external appearance of the nose.

In many cases, septoplasty is combined with rhinoplasty,
resulting in both functional *and* cosmetic improvement.

Years on antihistamines and headache medications
had done nothing to relieve Charley's chronic sinus problems. He was an allergic child, now thirty-two, and
afraid that he would have to quit his job at an auto body
shop. Paint and chemical fumes were taking their toll
and leaving him in almost constant discomfort.

No amount of medication could totally relieve these
symptoms, because, in addition to his allergies, Charley's
airways were obstructed by a severely deviated septum.
Even with his allergies under control, Charley still had
compromised airways.

As we discussed repairing his septum, Charley asked
me what his nose would look like. When I told him it
would look the same, he replied that, if he was going to
go through with the operation, he wanted "something to
show for it." Specifically, he wanted the hook in his nose

removed. He was tired of hearing jokes about his "honker."

Charley underwent septoplasty and rhinoplasty. For the entire ten days that the splint was on and the packing was in, he reported that he felt as if he had the worst al-

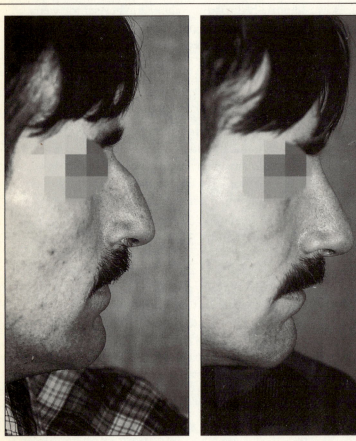

Rhinoplasty: Before, left, and six months after, right. Rhinoplasty to remove the hook in the nose was combined with septoplasty to correct a severely deviated septum.

lergy attack ever and looked like he had been mugged. He arrived an hour and a half early for his appointment to have his splint removed. Immediately, he was able to breathe better—he had never had so much air go through his nose at one time. In fact, he felt light-headed.

It was only after he adjusted to his new breathing ability that Charley was able to fully appreciate his new profile. The jokes are gone . . . but the paint smells even worse.

Definitions

Ala nasi   The outer wing-shaped wall of the nostril.

Alar cartilage   The connective tissue that makes up the tip of the nose.

Alar rim   The border of the nostril.

Nasal dorsum   The ridge of the nose formed of bone at the bridge and cartilage at the tip.

Nasal septum   The wall dividing the nasal cavity into halves, formed posteriorly of bone and anteriorly of cartilage.

Rhinoplasty   Reconstructive or plastic surgery of the nose.

Septoplasty   Reconstructive surgery of the nasal septum.

Rhinoplasty

The Procedure

This operation is designed to alter the external appearance of the nose. This may be done to modify an inherited characteristic or correct an acquired deformity.

Once you are asleep, the surgeon will usually place packing moistened with anesthetic into your nasal passages to numb the lining and constrict the blood vessels. The sensory nerves of the nose are then numbed with a local anesthetic. This serves to reduce intraoperative bleeding, postoperative bruising, and postoperative discomfort.

In the case of simple fracture of a nasal bone—for example, when one side of the nose is depressed—the broken fragment is manipulated back into place using a blunt instrument. No incisions are required.

As a rule, external incisions are avoided at all costs because of frequent complications with healing.

In more extensive procedures, incisions are placed inside the nostrils. In these, the dorsal hump may be reduced by rasping or removing a portion of the nasal bones. Widened or displaced bones may require fracturing so that they can be repositioned to achieve the desired contour. Finally, the alar cartilage is sculpted to refine the nasal tip. The incisions are closed with dissolving sutures. The nasal packing is removed, and then an external dressing of tape is applied. A splint is often utilized both to reduce swelling and to provide protection.

Septoplasty

The Procedure

This operation is designed to straighten a deviation of the nasal septum. The deviation may be genetic or it may have been acquired, secondary to trauma.

Once you are asleep, the surgeon will usually place packing moistened with anesthetic into your nasal passages to numb the lining and constrict the blood vessels. The sensory nerves of the nose are then numbed with a local anesthetic. This serves to reduce intraoperative bleeding, postoperative bruising, and postoperative discomfort.

Septoplasty incisions are also commonly placed inside the nostrils. Through these, the entire septum may be exposed so that deviated segments may be resected or reshaped, allowing for central positioning. Because the septum has a "mem-ory," there is a tendency for it to return to the deviated position. Packing is used to counteract this tendency and hold the septum in place during healing. The incisions are closed with dissolving sutures. An external dressing and splint are used, especially if septoplasty is combined with rhinoplasty.

Length of Procedure

Rhinoplasty requires one to one and one-half hours.
    Septoplasty requires one to one and one-half hours.
    Combined, the operation requires one and one half to two hours.

Anesthesia

You will be asleep, either under general anesthesia or sedation. In either case, topical and local anesthetics are utilized.

In/Outpatient

Rhinoplasty and septoplasty are almost always outpatient procedures. If general anesthesia is used, the operation will be done in a hospital on an outpatient basis.

Incisions/Scarring

Standard incisions are placed inside the nasal airways. There are no external scars unless a section of the alar rim is removed to narrow the nostrils. This leaves an external scar at the base of the alar rim. External incisions are generally avoided because of their tendency for poor cosmetic scars.

Pain

Rhinoplasty patients complain of the nuisance of wearing the splint and the inability to breathe easily through the nose rather than any specific pain. Medications are prescribed to relieve these symptoms.

Septoplasty patients find the packing, at best, a nuisance. Pain medication is used to take the edge off, but you will still count the days until the packing comes out.

Specific Risks

* During the initial healing phase, trauma to the nose may displace the nose and re-create the deformity.

* Some asymmetry is expected. Any significant imbalance may require a secondary operation.

Recovery Time

* Desk job: You will be allowed to return to work in three or four days; most people wait a full week to ten days to allow for splint removal.
* Manual labor: Bending, lifting heavy weights, or straining are restricted for at least one week. Your doctor will advise you.

Exercise
Most patients can resume their usual level of aerobic activity two to three weeks after the operation. Your doctor will advise you.

Sex
Same as for exercise. Wait for about a week. Don't try anything new or strenuous for a couple of weeks.

Sun
Stay out of the sun for the first week. Always use sunscreen and wear sunglasses.

Travel

There are no restrictions on travel by automobile, airplane, or bus.

Frequency/Duration of Results

Results are permanent. This is usually a one-time operation.

What to Expect

You will have an external, obvious dressing on your nose for a week to ten days.

During this time, you will breathe through your mouth. *Sleep in a room with a humidifier.*

Cold compresses are generally applied at frequent intervals for the first twenty-four hours to minimize bruising and swelling. *Frozen peas in a zip-top plastic bag wrapped in a hand towel make an excellent compress.*

After twenty-four hours, you may find that warm compresses help to resolve bruising and swelling. *Some patients prefer to continue cold compresses during this time; most find warm compresses beneficial.*

You will swallow some blood in the course of the operation. Do not be alarmed if your stools darken.

Start out with sips of clear, noncarbonated liquid. Make sure that your stomach is settled before resuming normal eating and drinking.

Expect two black eyes. You may or may not get them, but if you do, it takes a week to ten days for them to resolve.

You may find it more comfortable to tape your eyeglasses to your forehead for the first week or two rather than letting them rest on the bridge of your nose.

Expect to look worse before you look better. Prepare family—and especially small children—for this prior to having your operation.

You will look worse than you feel. Let those close to you know that this is part of the recovery process.

You will need to keep your head elevated at all times, including at night, for the first week, as this will reduce bruising and swelling. *A recliner will keep you in the proper position.*

You will be able to shower from the neck down and wash your hair beauty-parlor style, but you may not get your dressing wet.

Once the splint is removed, the nasal skin will be very dry and will require moisturizing. Your doctor will suggest something suitable for you.

It will take up to one year for total resolution of postoperative swelling to occur.

If the tip of your nose is numb after the operation, it will take several months for the feeling to return.

Fees/Insurance

Fees for primary nose reshaping are between $4,000 and $5,500 for open rhinoplasty; $3,800 and $4,500 for closed. Secondary rhinoplasty costs between $3,800 and $4,500 for open, and between $2,700 and $3,000 for closed.

Most insurance policies do not cover rhinoplasty when it is performed for a purely cosmetic purpose.

Fees for septoplasty begin at $3,500.

If you require septoplasty to correct breathing problems or rhinoplasty to correct a deformity caused either by a congenital defect or by an accident, you may qualify for insurance reimbursement. Consult your insurance carrier and secure written preauthorization. Your primary care physician and surgeon can advise you.

Important Questions to Ask About Rhinoplasty and Septoplasty

- ❖ Will I require any external incisions?

- ❖ Will the bones in my nose need to be broken?

- ❖ Will I have packing left in my nose?

- ❖ How long will the splint stay on?

- ❖ What is a realistic recovery time for me?

6

The Ears

~

❖ Otoplasty ❖ Ear Lobe Repair ❖ Ear Lobe Augmentation

While protruding ears, lop ears, and a variety of related congenital anomalies are not *life-threatening* physical disabili-
ties, the emotional toll is potentially devastating. Ideally,
correction is performed around the age of five, before the
child starts school. This will protect the child from the teas-
ing and tormenting of peers.

Most often, malformed ears are corrected in childhood,
but it is common for teenagers and adults to request it as
well.

Other plastic surgical procedures used to improve the appearance of one's ears include earlobe reduction and augmentation and repair of torn earlobes. These operations are
discussed on page 131.

Randi was a lively eighteen-year-old with lots of thick,
curly hair, so the fact that her ears stuck out had never
been an issue to her. However, she loved to swim and
hang out at the beach and pool. Her favorite activity,
swimming, exposed her most hated feature, her ears,
which stuck through her wet hair. The only solution
would have been to wear a bathing cap, which was too
uncool to be an option.

For her high school graduation present, Randi's parents financed the operation to correct the position of her
ears. Now she can wear her long hair any way she wants

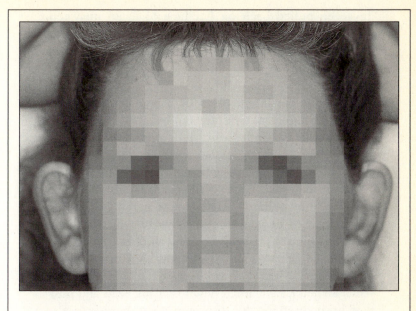

Otoplasty: Before, above, and one month postoperative, below.

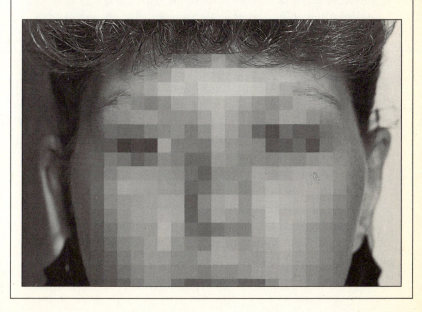

to—even pulled back off her face or in an upsweep, something she *never* would have done—and she can enjoy swimming without fear of being teased about her "Dumbo ears."

With one ear larger than the other, James was the brunt of a family joke throughout his childhood. Everyone said that, when he was a little boy, he had been so badly behaved that his mother was always pulling on his ear . . . and that she'd pulled so much that one was bigger than the other. Because his parents didn't consider this condition to be life-threatening, nothing was done about it when he was a child. Once he was out on his own, he found that his insurance wouldn't cover the operation and he didn't have the financial means to pay for it himself.

As an actor, he learned how to tilt his head and position his body so that his disproportionate ear was not so obvious, especially from a distance. However, up close, especially in photographs, James said that all he could see was his prominent ear. He was reminded of how he hated looking at his family photo album.

As soon as James was able to finance the operation, he had it done as an outpatient under local anesthesia. It was wintertime, so he wore the headband to protect his freshly repaired ear without being too conspicuous. After a week, he was able to return to his desk job and auditions without any obvious evidence. He continued to wear the headband at night for a month. At last he was able to get his hair, which he usually wore long and shaggy, cut into a more up-to-date style.

At last report, James had had a new set of head shots made and was sending them out to producers and casting directors.

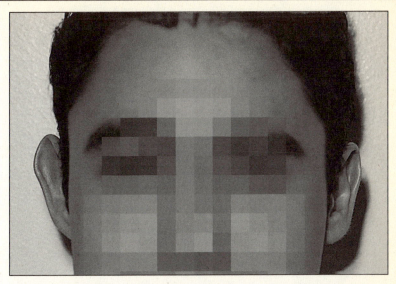

Unilateral Otoplasty: Before, above, and four months after having oto-plasty, below, to correct the size of one ear that was much larger than the other.

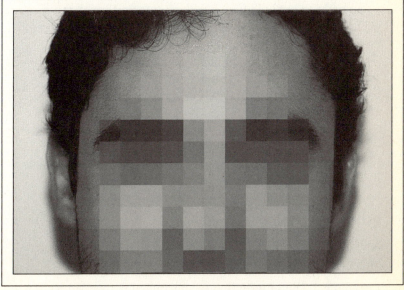

Otoplasty

Overview

Otoplasty is an operation to correct a condition that is almost always congenital. The classic ear deformity is caused by *unfurling of the antihelix* (the normal crease in the ear's cartilage). Another common problem is conchal cartilage excess—simply too much cartilage. All other congenital deformities are variations of these.

Frequently, these conditions are bilateral—affecting both ears—however, there are instances where one side is more prominent than the other.

Ears may also be damaged by impact. Bleeding effectively kills cartilage, causing the outer ear to become knotted and gnarled, hence the nickname, cauliflower ear. Intervention to stop bleeding at the time of injury is the ideal treatment protocol; however, this may not be sufficient to prevent deformity. Surgical repair is possible at any age.

Something as obvious as one's ears sticking out or flopping over can be an emotionally charged issue, one that is corrected relatively simply in the hands of an able plastic surgeon.

The operation in young children is usually performed before they start school. By this age, their bodies are better able to tolerate general anesthesia. Older children and adults usually have the procedure done under local anesthesia alone.

Incisions are placed on the back side of the ear where they will be difficult to see. Most of the time, they are covered by hair. Boys tend to have their ears corrected sooner than girls because of shorter hairstyles.

Definitions

Antihelix   The inner fold in the cartilage that gives the outer ear its shape.

Cartilage   The connective tissue (gristle) that forms the outer ear.

Cauliflower ears   An acquired deformity of the ear, also known as boxer's ear, caused by injury.

Conchal cartilage excess   A congenital condition in which there is too much cartilage in the lower portion of the ear, making the base of the ear stick out.

Lop ear deformity   A congenital condition in which the top of the ear flops forward, resulting from an unfurling of the antihelix. Also known as rabbit ears.

Otoplasty   A medical term referring to the surgical correction of an ear deformity.

The Procedure

The purpose of this operation is to re-create the anatomical folds of the cartilage. This may or may not involve removal of cartilage, but it almost always involves carving and suturing the cartilage.

An incision is made on the back of the ear to expose the cartilage so that it can be sculpted or folded, as mandated by the degree of deformity and type of correction. Occasionally, a piece of cartilage will be removed to provide a more natural-looking fold. Another technique calls for removal of skin. Sutures are used to fold the cartilage back on itself to reshape the ear without cartilage removal. Permanent sutures may be used to maintain the new shape.

Variations on this basic procedure may be applied to correct a wide variety of outer-ear deformities.

Length of Procedure

Ear operations usually take forty-five minutes per ear.

Anesthesia

You and your doctor have two options, influenced primarily by your wishes or, in the case of children, their age.

Local   For most adults and older children, injections of local anesthetic to numb the ear and surrounding tissue are usually sufficient for most otoplasty procedures.

Local plus Sedation   Some patients may prefer sedation plus local anesthetic. Your doctor will advise you of the pros and cons of each.

General Anesthesia   This is usually reserved for young children.

In/Outpatient

Otoplasty is usually performed as an outpatient procedure in a hospital or ambulatory surgical facility.

Incisions/Scarring

Because the incision is usually made in the back of the ear, concealment is not a major concern. *Let your hair grow before your operation to assist in camouflage.*

Take care to protect the ears from trauma for four to six weeks, as this can tear the sutures that are holding the cartilage in place before healing is completed which could recreate the deformity. Once the ear is completely healed you don't have to worry about that.

Pain

Adequate padding and dressing usually limits postoperative discomfort. In fact, severe pain after otoplasty can be an indication of bleeding, which requires immediate attention as bleeding effectively kills cartilage. This will result in a condition known as cauliflower ear or boxer's ear.

Any soreness or discomfort is easily managed with acetaminophen or some other over-the-counter analgesic.

Specific Risks

❖ In rare cases, a patient can develop an infection in the cartilage, which can cause scar tissue to form. Usually, such
infections are treated successfully with antibiotics. In difficult cases, an operation may be required to drain the infected area or remove the infected cartilage.

❖ Fluid or blood accumulation under the skin usually produces intense pain and requires immediate drainage by
your surgeon.

❖ Trauma to the newly repaired ear can produce bleeding or
even re-create the deformity. A cauliflower ear deformity
may result if this is untreated.

Recovery Time

Return to Work:
❖ Desk job or school: If you can work with the dressing on,
you can return to work the next day. Otherwise, you must
wait for dressing removal. Avoid any activity in which the
ear might be bent or hit for a month or so.
❖ Manual labor: Avoid bending, lifting, or straining for at
least two weeks. Follow your doctor's advice.

Exercise
With a protective bandage, like a headband, you should be
increasing your activity level at a steady pace, avoiding contact sports, with no restrictions by four weeks.

Most patients resume their usual level of aerobic activity
a week after the operation. Avoid any activity in which the
ear could be bent or hit. Do nothing strenuous without your
doctor's permission.

Sex
Same as for exercise. Wait for about a week. Avoid anything that involves direct physical contact with the ears.

Sun
Stay out of the sun for the first week. Always use sunscreen to protect scars.

Travel
There are no restrictions on travel.

Frequency/Duration of Results

Results are permanent.

What to Expect

Immediately after the operation, your head will be wrapped in a bulky, turbanlike bandage to promote the best molding and healing.

After four or five days, these bulky bandages will be replaced by a lighter dressing, like a headband. Your surgeon will give you directions for wearing this, especially at night so that you won't do any damage if you toss and turn in your sleep.

Children need to wear more substantial bandages because of play and, for this reason, they may wear heavier bandages for longer. Adults may get by with only a headband during sleep. *An adult may want to schedule this operation in the wintertime when wearing a headband won't be so conspicuous.*

There may be bruising when the bandage is first taken off, but this generally resolves within a week.

This procedure is relatively pain free unless you hit the ear or put pressure on it. This is significant for people who use the telephone a lot. *If it is not possible for you to limit telephone use, get a speaker phone.*

Fees/Insurance

The usual surgeon's fee for this procedure is $3,500 to $5,000 for correction of both ears, slightly less for one.

Frequently, this procedure is covered by insurance if performed on children. It is more difficult to obtain coverage for adults.

Important Questions to Ask About Otoplasty

- ❖ Where will the scar be?

- ❖ Can I hide the scars with my present hairstyle? *(Keep your hair long enough to cover your ears for the first month after your operation.)*

- ❖ When can I wash my hair? *(If you chemically treat your hair, you'd better do it just before your operation since you won't be able to do anything about it for a month because the chemicals may adversely affect the new scar.)*

- ❖ How long will I need to wear a bandage?

- ❖ What is a realistic recovery timetable for me?

- ❖ Will I be able to wear my glasses while my ears are healing?

Earlobe Procedures

Earlobe Repair

It is not uncommon that people with pierced ears who wear large or heavy earrings may, over time, experience stretched holes as well as the earlobes themselves. In some people, this hole is stretched so much that it no longer can contain a post-type earring. In others, usually at the hands of an inquisitive baby, an earring is ripped completely through the lobe, leaving a bifid, or forked, earlobe.

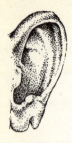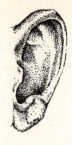

Correction of Ear Lobe Tear: Left, before repair. Right, the rim of the tear is excised and the edges sewn together to close the tear.

Repair of a partially or completely torn lobe is performed under local anesthesia in the doctor's office. In each case, the torn rim of the defect is excised and the edges are sewn together. Sutures are usually removed in seven to ten days, and you are left with a scar that looks like a crease in the earlobe.

Usually, after four to six weeks, repiercing can be done, *but not in exactly the same place.* The reason for this is that the scar is not strong enough to support earrings, and you will be likely to develop another tear if the same area is used.

Fees and Insurance

Cost of repairing of the earlobes is between $600 and $750 per ear. It is unlikely that this will be covered by insurance unless the tear occurred as part of an otherwise covered accident or crime.

Earlobe Reduction/Augmentation

A minor but troublesome problem in some patients is the progressive enlargement of the earlobes, with or without thinning. They complain that their earlobes have become long and floppy, making it difficult for them to wear their favorite earrings.

Earlobe reduction is done in a similar manner as earlobe repair, discussed above.

For thinning lobes, fat grafts add bulk to the lobe. See chapter 11, page 206.

7

The Head and Neck

~

❖ Face- and Neck-Lift ❖ Forehead- and Brow-Lift

Have you ever noticed that, when the conversation turns to plastic surgery, at least one person will raise their fingers to their temples and push the skin back in a parody of a face-lift? That's because this is one of the most known—and notorious—of all cosmetic operations.

The earliest face-lift procedures—when it seemed that only movie stars and wealthy widows had them—tightened the skin alone to take away wrinkles. They had the potential of creating a too-tight, masklike look. Today, thanks to advanced surgical techniques, a more natural appearance is achieved by restoring sagging muscles to their original positions as well as resecting excess skin.

Plastic surgeons divide the face into three aesthetic units. They treat the first unit, the forehead, with a brow-lift. The second and third units, the face and neck, though visually separated, are anatomically linked and are approached simultaneously in what is commonly known as a face-lift operation. Eyelids are corrected separately. (Eyelid procedures are discussed in chapter 4.)

The profile of patients requesting face-lifts is changing. Not only are women considering face-lifts at a younger age, but also more than ever, men are seeking the procedure.

No matter how little or how much work the neck needs, it is corrected in the same operation as the face, while brow-

or forehead-lifts may be done independently of any other facial procedure.

Your surgeon will recommend having one procedure over the other, depending upon the degree of your problem, and the time you have available for recovery. Make sure that you are clear in your understanding of which procedures apply to you.

Definitions

Brow ptosis   Sagging of the eyebrow below the level of the upper rim of the eye socket.

Composite or deep plane face-lift   An extensive face-lift procedure that involves dissection of all layers of the facial soft tissues.

Glabellar Frown Lines   The vertical creases between the eyebrows.

Jowls   A term used to describe lax skin and pockets of fat that blunt the jawline.

Marionette lines   A term used to describe vertical creases extending from the corners of the mouth to the jaw.

Nasolabial fold   The crease extending from the side of the nostril to the corner of the mouth.

Platysmal bands   Cords of the platysma muscle (the anterior superficial neck muscle), which extend from the jaw to the collarbone on either side of the neck.

Rhytid   A wrinkle.

Rhytidectomy   The surgical procedure to remove wrinkles; a face-lift.

SMAS (submusculo aponeurotic segment) face-lift   A two-tiered face-lift procedure, the major component of which is tightening of the connective tissue and muscular layer of the face before redraping the skin.

Submental fat The fat found under the chin, commonly associated with double chins.

Tragus A tonguelike projection of cartilage in front of the opening of the ear canal.

Face- and Neck-Lift (Rhytidectomy)

Overview

Early face-lift operations tightened only the skin, placing *all* of the tension on the suture line. This stress frequently widened the scars, making them and, indeed, the face-lift itself very obvious. Since the skin has an amazing capacity for expansion, results were not only less than optimal, they were also short-lived. Patients who had this procedure repeated too quickly often developed that telltale, overdone mask.

With a better understanding of anatomy, the tension in a face-lift operation has been transferred to the deeper anatomic layers. The most common procedure today involves tightening of the SMAS layer—the submusculo aponeurotic segment—with redraping of the skin.

A newer, less widely accepted but widely debated extension of this technique is the deep plane face-lift. Considerably more invasive than the SMAS face-lift, this technique distributes the tension through *all* layers of the facial soft tissue, right down to the bone.

Regardless of the technique, while one may concentrate in one area more than the other, face- and neck-lifts are usually done at the same time. By *face*, we mean the lower two-thirds of the face, i.e., from the eyes down. A face-lift alone will not improve the wrinkles across the upper lip (see chapter 8) nor will it address eyelid problems (see chapter 4).

Janet was concerned that, at forty-two, she was losing credibility as an image consultant. Despite meticulous skin care, diet and exercise, she had a general laxity of her facial muscles and skin, resulting in a loss of jaw and neckline definition, and deepening of her nasal labial lines. She came to me to find out if anything could be done to improve her appearance. She feared that, if she had a significant face-lift *now*, she would be doomed to a lifetime of repeat face-lifts.

I told her that, indeed, she *could* wait ten to fifteen years before having anything done, but that if she did, her condition would be worse, requiring more extensive

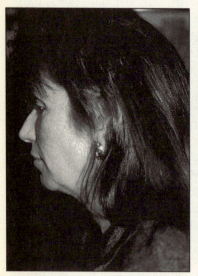 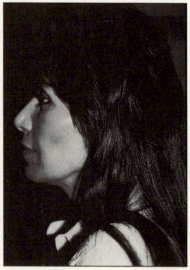

Face-lift: Left, woman in her early 40's before a face-lift. Right, three months after the procedure, she looks fresher, healthier and more relaxed, if not necessarily younger. By having work done at this age there is more good tissue to work with, and this patient can expect easier healing and longer-lasting results than a similar procedure done on an older patient.

procedures and making for a more obvious change. In truth, Janet's skin and muscle tone would never be better than they were now. Treatment at this time would actually serve as intervention—maintenance versus reconstruction—allowing for a less extensive operation in terms of muscle tightening and redraping of skin.

Janet had a multilayered face-lift, which repositioned facial muscles back over her cheekbones. This restored definition to her cheeks. Fat under her chin was removed by liposuction and her neck muscles were tightened. This was done at the start of a two-week vacation. She was able to return to work right on schedule with only a little adaptation in her makeup for camouflage. Rather than looking younger, she reported that she felt that she looked like a well-rested forty-two-year old.

Less invasive facial surgery done at a younger age will not halt aging. It does, however, produce longer-lasting results. While Janet may want to have minor touch-up procedures at intervals in the future to maintain the effect, it would be unlikely that she must undergo a complete face-lift again as long as she continues her current skin-care and health and fitness programs.

The Procedure

There are multiple variations of the face-lift technique. In most cases, a face-lift is performed while you are asleep. Sedation is used much more commonly than general anesthesia. A local anesthetic containing epinephrine is usually injected to numb the area of the dissection and to reduce intraoperative bleeding and postoperative discomfort.

The traditional incisions are placed behind the temporal hairline, above and slightly in front of the ear, then extended downward in a natural line in front of the ear to the earlobe (or just behind the tragus, the cartilage at the front of the outer ear) and around to the back of the ear and into the lower posterior scalp. If the neck muscles need to be tightened and/or platysmal bands corrected, a small incision under the chin will be added.

Despite the fact that incisions are designed to be hidden by hair or to follow natural skin folds, hair is not usually shaved for this operation. Instead, hair is parted and secured out of the way.

After the skin is then dissected off the muscle layer, various techniques can be used to elevate the sagging muscles. These include simple plication, or pleating, of the SMAS layer, in much the same way as a tailor makes a dart in a piece of fabric. Another variation involves lifting the margins of the SMAS layer, cutting away any excess, and suturing it into its newly elevated position. Finally, in the most invasive face-lift procedure, the dissection at the surface of the facial bones elevates all of the soft tissues. Think of this as repairing the infrastructure of a building before painting it.

Frequently, liposuction techniques are used to remove excess fat and sculpt bony landmarks, such as the jawline.

After this is completed, the skin is redraped, and the excess is removed. The skin is sutured *without* tension, to ensure the finest scars possible. Frequently, some form of compression dressing is applied.

Length of Procedure

A face-lift takes about three hours to perform.

Anesthesia

Most face-lift procedures are performed under sedation or under general anesthesia. In either case, a local anesthetic with epinephrine is also used to decrease intraoperative bleeding and reduce postoperative discomfort.

In/Outpatient

Face-lifts are outpatient procedures. Some facilities provide for overnight nursing care; others send patients home with professional nursing care.

Pain

Prescription pain medication is required for the first several days.

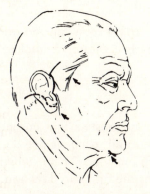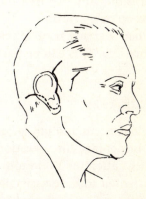

Standard Face-lift Incisions: Left, the incisions for face lifts are usually placed where they can be easily camouflaged by the hair or fall into natural skin folds. Traditionally, incisions are placed behind the temporal hairline, above and slightly in front of the ear, then extended downward in a natural line in front of the ear to the ear lobe (or just behind the tragus, the cartilage at the front of the outer ear) and around to the back of the ear and into the lower posterior scalp. If the neck muscles need to be tightened and/or platysmal bands corrected, a small incision under the chin will be added. Right, frequently liposuction is used to remove excess fat and sculpt bony landmarks, such as the jawline. After this is completed, the skin is redraped and the excess removed. The skin is sutured without tension to ensure the finest scars possible.

Incisions/Scarring

There are several variations of incision placement. Ideally, incisions are positioned where they will be hidden by hair or fall into natural skin folds. The most difficult incisions for the patient to manage are those placed along the hairline, giving it an unnatural sharpness, particularly noticeable when hair is worn short or upswept.

Healing scars are easily covered with hair or a beard, which is a primary reason to let your hair grow before your operation. Any exposed incisions can be easily hidden by makeup or a beard.

Poor scarring usually results from excess tension on the suture line. This can be particularly common in smokers.

Specific Risks

❖ Fluid accumulation is one of the most serious complications of face-lift operations. It usually occurs when the patient attempts to do too much too soon. This is why it is *essential* to have assistance for the first two days and follow a realistic, gradual return to normal activity under the direction of your doctor.

❖ Poor scarring and/or skin loss is a significant risk in patients who smoke. *Many surgeons will not do face-lifts on patients who smoke. If you intend to stop smoking, you must do it at least two weeks before the operation as it takes this long to clear the system of the toxins.* **This is serious. Don't put yourself at unnecessary risk by lying to your surgeon. If you smoke, fess up.**

❖ Temporary alteration of skin sensation is common. Permanent alteration is rare.

❖ Temporary paralysis of facial muscles, particularly in the bottom lip area, is rare. Permanent paralysis is even rarer.

❖ Skin irregularities, such as dimpling, rippling, bagginess, or asymmetry are frequent but seldom permanent. If they persist, they can usually be corrected quite easily with a second limited procedure to smooth out the skin.

❖ Pigmentation changes may become permanent if incisions are exposed to the sun soon after the operation.

❖ Hair loss, usually in the temporal region, is a response to excess tension along the suture line. It can take as long as three months for hair regrowth to begin. If permanent loss occurs, a hair restoration procedure may be indicated.

Recovery Time

Return to Work
Realistically, you will not feel up to returning to work of any kind for the better part of a week. One's energy level does not usually return to normal for four to six weeks. It is important to plan your life accordingly.

By the second week, with the help of camouflage, most people are able to return to a desk job.

Manual labor, or work that requires you to be on your feet for most of the day, should be done only under the direction of your doctor.

Exercise
Begin walking around as soon as comfort allows to stimulate circulation and promote healing. Many short walks rather than one long one are the best exercise during the first week.

Once bruising has disappeared, increase your level of activity according to your doctor's protocol.

Sex
You may want to take it easy during the first week. Don't try anything strenuous for a couple of weeks.

Sun

Stay out of the sun for the first week. Wide-brimmed, floppy hats with ties are advised to protect the face and incisions.

Travel

There are no restrictions on travel by automobile, airplane, or bus. You may not feel up to extended travel for about a week.

Frequency/Duration of Results

Results are *not* permanent. One of the most commonly asked questions about any face-lift is, "How long will it last?" The answer depends on the state of the tissues involved at the time of the operation. In general, younger tissues hold the lift longer.

Newer operations that involve muscle tightening will last longer than procedures that tighten only the skin. Remember that a face-lift *resets* your biological clock; it doesn't stop it. At some point, your face will be back where you started.

As a face-lift starts to loosen, smaller touch-up procedures will extend the life of your lift. It is not necessary to go through the entire procedure all over again if intermittent steps are taken.

Needless to say, large fluctuations in weight, tobacco or alcohol use, and exposure to the sun adversely affect your lift. Other plastic surgery procedures, such as chemical peels, may prolong the life of your lift.

It is these variables that make it difficult if not impossible to precisely determine the life span of your lift.

What to Expect

You will need assistance for the first forty-eight hours as bending, lifting, and straining must be avoided. By two days after your operation, you should be able to take care of yourself.

The first two days are the most difficult. It is during this time that pain medication is used liberally.

Dull, aching pain is to be expected. Sharp pain on only one side may be an indication of a problem. If this occurs, contact your doctor immediately.

You will need to keep your head elevated at all times, including at night, for the first week as this will reduce bruising and swelling. *A recliner will keep you in the proper position.*

There will be some blood in your hair, so put an old towel on your pillow to prevent staining.

Expect to look worse before you look better. Prepare family—and especially small children—for this prior to having your operation.

You will look worse than you feel. Let those close to you know that this is part of the recovery process.

If a *compression* bandage is used, it is usually removed after two days. If a *support* bandage, like that used in liposuction procedures, is used, it is worn for a longer period. Take it off to shower and wash. Follow your doctor's instructions.

Most doctors allow their rhidectomy patients to shower and gently wash their hair after two days. Use *tepid* water and mild shampoo.

Men should avoid shaving for the first postoperative week if at all possible.

Your neck will feel very stiff and you will feel like you can't turn your head. This is due to postoperative swelling. There is no advantage in trying to stretch out the tension at this point.

Men may need to shave *behind* their ears initially due to the advancement of their beard lines and may want to consider electrolysis or other permanent hair removal once healing is completed.

You probably will **not** like the way you look for four to six weeks.

You will start to look your best at three to six months.

You should expect a change in sensation, usually numbness, in your skin right after the procedure. It takes about three months for full sensation to return.

Unevenness will be present. This is usually caused by swelling and will resolve over the first four to six weeks. *Dramatic differences from one side to the other may indicate bleeding under the skin and should be reported to your doctor immediately.*

Expect to feel some lumps under your skin. These are localized areas of bruising. Your body will absorb them over two to four weeks.

Expect a period of the blues. This occurs, usually two to three weeks after your operation, at a time when you are not feeling or looking your very best. This will pass . . . and it will pass more quickly when you realize what it is.

Be aware that you will not be able to chemically treat your hair for one month after your operation. *It is recommended that you color, perm, or straighten your hair beforehand. Also, let your hair grow longer before your operation so that it can camouflage your incisions while they heal.*

Expect that you won't feel up to par for *at least* six weeks. It will take this long for you to regain your energy level. Plan your business and social schedules accordingly.

Fees/Insurance

The usual cost of face- and neck-lifts ranges from $7,500 to $16,000.

This procedure is not usually covered by insurance.

Important Questions to Ask About Face-Lifts

❖ How many scars will there be?

❖ Where will the scars be? Will they affect how I style my hair?

- ◆ Will my head be shaved?

- ◆ Will I need nursing care?

- ◆ What kind of bandage or dressing will be used?

- ◆ Will I need a compression garment, and what will it look like?

- ◆ What is a realistic recovery timetable for me?

Forehead- and Brow-Lift

Overview

A lift of the forehead or brow reduces wrinkles in the top third of the face—from the eyebrows upward. If it is to be done with upper eyelid plasty, it must be done *first* to avoid overcorrection of the eye-lift. Such overcorrection could leave a patient with a "surprised" look or worse, an inability to close the eyes completely.

A brow-lift alone will not improve the wrinkled or sagging lower eyelids (see chapter 4).

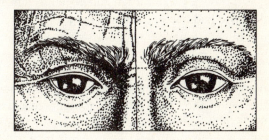

Brow-Lift: Before correction, left, the lines over and between the brows are deep. Often this is exacerbated by low-hanging eyebrows, giving an intense, often unfriendly appearance. The forehead muscles responsible for these creases are released and raised to create a more open, approachable brow line, right.

Robert was suffering a midlife crisis as he approached his fortieth birthday. A highly successful manager of an upscale men's store, he was concerned that his job was in jeopardy, since his regional manager had recently told him that he always looked angry and that he intimidated people, especially the people working under him. At our first meeting, Robert told me, "Basically, I'm a nice guy, but people think I'm a real S.O.B. until they get to know me."

On examination, I noted that he not only had deep creases in his forehead and glabellar frown lines between his brows but he also had eyebrows that hung low. This gave him an intense, unpleasant appearance.

Even though his wife thought he was crazy to want to do anything, Robert went ahead and scheduled his operation in late February. He told his colleagues and children that he was going on a fishing trip. This allowed him time to recuperate in private at his family's summer house. He returned from his trip a week later, looking rested and refreshed, with the swelling and bruising resolved and the incision covered by his hair.

In the office, Robert was smiling and almost jovial. He looked as though a great burden had been lifted from his shoulders. He had become approachable.

The Procedure

Traditionally, a brow-lift is performed using an incision that crosses the top of the head from ear to ear (see illustration, page 148). Hair is parted and the incision is made. (This is an operation suitable only for those who have a full head of hair, as it is used to cover the incision.)

For patients who are bald or have thinning hair, the incisions may be placed just above each eyebrow. This, too, is not without drawbacks as it puts the scar in a potentially obvious place and can result in eyebrow distortion or even permanent loss. Another alternative for the balding patient involves use of the endoscopic approach as discussed in chapter 11.

Through the standard incision, the scalp and forehead skin are elevated at the level of the skull. Once the attachment of the brows to the skull is released, they are transposed superiorly, or raised, without extensive scalp resection.

Another important step is the weakening of overactive forehead muscles responsible for causing creases between the brows and forehead. This procedure has largely replaced an older technique involving resection, or removal of the overactive muscles, which often led to permanent nerve damage and contour irregularities.

Usually, no dressing is applied to the incision.

Length of Procedure

A brow-lift operation usually takes one and a half to two hours.

Anesthesia

Most brow-lift procedures are performed under sedation or under general anesthesia. In either case, a local anesthetic with epinephrine is also used to decrease intraoperative bleeding and reduce postoperative discomfort.

In/Outpatient

Brow-lifts are outpatient procedures.

Incisions/Scarring

The scalp incision leaves a permanent scar, which is totally within the standard hairline where it will be hidden. If you do lose your hair, it will be seen.

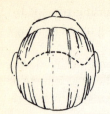

Incision for Brow-Lift: Traditionally, the incision for a brow-lift is positioned well within the hairline, where it will be hidden. It will start high at the temple and, following a W pattern, across the top of the head. Patients who have high foreheads or thinning hair have the options of having incisions placed along the upper margins of each eyebrow or using an endoscope to place multiple small incisions within the scalp.

Poor scarring may result if excess tension is placed on the suture line. Smokers are in a category by themselves and run an increased risk for poor scarring because of compromised circulation and retarded wound healing.

In patients with high foreheads or thinning hair, there are two options: The first is placement of incisions along the upper margins of each eyebrow, and the second requires multiple small incisions with the use of the endoscope, as described in chapter 11.

Pain

Prescription pain medications may be used for the first two days. After that, over-the-counter pain medications may be used as required.

Specific Risks

- Poor scarring and/or skin loss is a significant risk in patients who smoke. *If you intend to stop smoking, you must do it at least two weeks before the operation as it takes this long to clear the system of the toxins.* **This is serious. Don't put yourself at unnecessary risk by lying to your surgeon.**

- Temporary alteration of skin sensation is common. Permanent alteration is rare.

✦ Permanent alteration of skin sensation is possible when too many of the overactive forehead muscles are resected instead of simply weakened.

✦ Contour irregularities, specifically depressions, are possible when too many of the overactive forehead muscles are resected instead of simply weakened.

✦ If a brow-lift is done in conjunction with upper eyelid plasty, it must be done *first* to avoid overcorrection in the eye-lift.

✦ If a nerve is cut in the process of releasing the muscles that cause wrinkling, paralysis can result and make it impossible for your to raise your eyebrows.

✦ Hair loss is a response to excess tension along the suture line. It can take as long as three months for hair regrowth to begin. If permanent loss occurs, a hair restoration procedure may be indicated.

Recovery Time

Return to Work
✦ Desk job: You'll be able to return to work after three or four days.
✦ Manual labor: You will be able to return to work after a week. Bending, lifting, or straining are restricted until your doctor gives the go-ahead.

Exercise
Many short walks are the best exercise during the first week. Once bruising has disappeared, increase your level of activity according to your doctor's protocol.

Sex
You may want to take it easy during the first week.

Sun

Stay out of the sun for the first week. Wide-brimmed, floppy hats with ties are advised to protect healing incisions.

Travel

There are no restrictions on travel by automobile, airplane, or bus. You may not feel up to extended travel for two to three days.

Frequency/Duration of Results

Results are relatively permanent. This is not an operation that is usually repeated.

What to Expect

The standard incision is across the top of the scalp. *If you run a risk of baldness, you should discuss alternatives of incision placement with your doctor, since scars will be evident.*

Your head will not be shaved. Instead, hair will be parted and secured out of the way during the operation.

Be aware that you will not be able to chemically treat your hair for one month after your operation. *It is recommended that you color, perm, or straighten your hair beforehand. Also, let your hair grow longer before your operation so that it can camouflage your incisions while they heal.*

Most doctors allow their brow-lift and face-lift patients to shower and gently wash their hair after two days. Use tepid water and mild shampoo.

You may or may not get black eyes. If you do, they take a week to resolve. Bruising is not as severe as in blepharoplasty.

Sutures usually need to be removed at seven to ten days after the operation.

You may have decreased sensation in the scalp that may take as long as three months to resolve. *Take precautions not to burn yourself when you use a hair dryer, electric rollers, curling irons, etc.*

There may be some degree of overcorrection due to post-operative swelling immediately after your operation. When this swelling subsides, this will be resolved.

The first two days are the most difficult. It is during this time that pain medication is used liberally.

Dull, aching pain is to be expected. Sharp pain may be an indication of a problem. If this occurs, contact your doctor immediately.

You will need to keep your head elevated at all times, including at night, for the first week, as this will reduce bruising and swelling. *A recliner will keep you in the proper position.*

There will be some blood in your hair, so put an old towel on your pillow to prevent staining.

Expect to look worse for about five days before you look better. Prepare family—and especially small children—for this prior to having your operation.

Fees/Insurance

The usual cost of a brow-lift ranges from $3,000 to $5,000.

This procedure is not usually covered by insurance.

Important Questions to Ask About Brow-Lifts

❖ How many scars will there be?

❖ Where will the scars be? Will they affect how I style my hair?

❖ Will my head be shaved?

❖ What kind of bandage or dressing will be used?

❖ Will I need nursing care?

8

Cosmetic Skin Resurfacing and Scar Revision

~

❖ Dermabrasion ❖ Chemical Peels ❖ Scar Repair Techniques ❖ Sclerotherapy ❖ Tattoo Removal

The skin is the largest organ of the body and, as such, merits its own medical specialist, the dermatologist. The dermatologist is a medical doctor, concerned primarily with the diagnosis and nonsurgical management of disorders of the skin such as rashes, acne, and eczema.

While many dermatologists are trained in surgical techniques, the plastic surgeon is frequently called upon to manage surgical problems of the skin, such as scars, large skin cancers, and tumors of the skin. Often, chemical peels or dermabrasion are done in conjunction with other cosmetic and reconstructive procedures.

This overlap of specialties accounts for some of the confusion expressed by patients who seek treatment for various skin disorders. A qualified dermatologist will know when to refer you to a plastic surgeon and vice versa. If you are unsure of where to start, your primary care physician will be able to advise you.

In this chapter, we will discuss cosmetic resurfacing of the skin as well as some of the techniques used to improve the appearance and placement of scars. The more investigational technologies, such as laser resurfacing, are discussed in chapter 11.

Skin resurfacing techniques are often used in tandem with other plastic surgery procedures such as face-lifts.

For years, Sylvia has spent her winters in Florida, taking full advantage of the warmer climate to play golf five times a week, doing the same thing tirelessly all summer at home near Philadelphia. Also, she had stopped smoking ten years ago, but she had smoked for more than thirty years. At sixty-two, she came to me wanting a face-lift.

While I advised her that she would benefit from a face-lift, the smoker's lines around her mouth would be unaffected by the procedure. Sylvia was afraid of having a chemical peel but agreed to dermabrasion of her upper lip, which was done at the same time as her face-lift.

Definitions

Alphahydroxy acids (AHAs)   The mildest of the chemical peel formulas, alphahydroxy acids include glycolic, lactic, fruit acids, etc. They are used to improve skin texture but are of limited value in treatment of deep wrinkles, uneven pigmentation, and scars.

Chemical peel   A nonspecific term used to describe chemabrasion by any of a wide variety of agents that remove the superficial layer(s) of the skin in a controlled fashion. The result is a smoother, more evenly textured, and more evenly pigmented skin surface.

Dermabrasion   A technique of mechanical buffing of the skin, much like the sanding of a piece of wood, to remove the superficial layer(s) of the skin in a controlled fashion. This procedure is generally reserved for more serious skin problems such as severe acne scarring and may be combined with a chemical peel or other plastic surgery procedures. The result is a smoother, more evenly textured, and more evenly pigmented skin surface.

Dermaplaning   A technique to remove superficial skin in layers using a dermatome, a mechanical device much like an electric razor. This is reserved for more serious skin problems, such as scars from major burns.

Excision   The act of cutting out. A surgical procedure to totally remove a tumor or scar.

Hydroquinone   A prescription bleaching agent, commonly used with Retin-A or AHA treatments for management of irregularities in skin pigmentation.

Hypertrophic scar   A medical term used to describe a widened or enlarged scar that remains within the boundaries of the initial injury or incision.

Keloid scar   A hypertrophic scar that has outgrown the boundaries of the initial injury. This occurs when the body continues to manufacture collagen after a wound has healed. The keloid scar, frequently itchy, is often redder, thicker, and harder than surrounding skin.

Milia   Cysts that look like whiteheads, which may form in a resurfaced area. Treatment requires unroofing or shaving off the top of the cyst so that it heals itself.

Phenol   The strongest of the chemical solutions, phenol produces a deep peel and is best used to treat patients with coarse facial wrinkles and/or extensive environmental skin damage, i.e., sun, chemical pollutants, tobacco, alcohol, etc.

Retin-A   A prescription medication derived from vitamin A, prescribed commonly by dermatologists in the treatment of acne and used frequently as an exfoliating pretreatment for chemical peels. Its therapeutic effect beyond acne control is stimulation of skin growth, resulting in smoother, healthier-appearing skin.

Scar   The connective tissue remnant of the body's healing process in response to injury.

Scar revision   A term used to describe a variety of procedures, including chemical peels, injections of steroids, or surgical revisions used to improve the appearance and/or orientation of scars.

Trichloroacetic acid (TCA) Most commonly used for medium-depth peeling, TCA is commonly used to treat fine surface wrinkles, uneven pigmentation, and superficial blemishes.

W-Plasty; Z-Plasty Common surgical techniques used to reorient scars so that they more closely conform to natural skin lines and creases, making them less noticeable. The letters describe the incision pattern.

Dermabrasion

Overview

Dermabrasion is the grandfather of all skin-smoothing procedures.

Learning from the skinned knees of childhood, pioneers in plastic surgery experimented in creating a *controlled injury* on rough, scarred, and otherwise irregular skin. The skin is treated with an abrading instrument to sand away the damaged outer layers. Once healed, the skin is smoother and pink, with many wrinkles reduced.

Although dermabrasion has been largely replaced by chemical peel procedures, it still has a place as an important skin resurfacing procedure, especially in cases of severe scarring. It is also a means of tattoo removal.

Best used on the face, dermabrasion is of limited value in other areas because of the unpredictability of skin healing.

The Procedure

Step 1: Pretreatment
If the procedure is being done on a patient with acne, it is imperative that all active eruptions be under control. There can be no open lesions.

Step 2: Preparation
All skin care and cosmetic products, including makeup and after-shave, are stopped twenty-four to forty-eight hours prior to the procedure.

Step 3: Degreasing
The skin is thoroughly cleansed with alcohol or acetone immediately prior to the procedure to remove all residue.

Step 4: Anesthesia
If a small area is to be treated, a local anesthetic is sufficient. For a larger area, a brief general anesthetic is used.

Step 5: Dermabrasion
Using any of a variety of abrading wheels, the surgeon planes and contours the irregular skin surface, feathering the margins of the area to avoid a masklike appearance.

Care is taken to monitor the depth of this abrasion to avoid deep injury that may cause additional scarring. For the first day or two, plasma oozes from the treated surface and forms a *coagulum,* or crust. This is not to be confused with *eschar,* or scab formation.

Step 6: Dressings and Immediate Aftercare
An antibiotic moisturizing ointment that serves as dressing is applied to all treated areas. These areas are cleansed with tepid water and fresh ointment is applied, usually two to three times a day, to avoid a crust buildup.

Step 7: Recovery and Maintenance
New skin has usually resurfaced the treated area within seven to ten days.

The treated area requires conscientious moisturizing and sunscreen protection. You will be sensitive to extremes of temperature and will notice a change in color when exposed to extreme temperatures for as long as a year following dermabrasion.

Depending upon the severity of contour irregularities, additional dermabrasion may be required. Wait from six to nine months for subsequent dermabrasion. Patients tolerate multiple superficial dermabrasions better than one deep procedure.

Length of Procedure

A full-face dermabrasion under general anesthesia requires thirty minutes.

In/Outpatient

A small area may be dermabraded in your doctor's office. Larger areas require use of a general anesthetic, which is administered in a hospital on an outpatient basis.

Incisions/Scarring

There are no incisions.

Pain

Dermabrasion creates a raw skin surface. The degree of pain is related to the depth of the abrasion. In most instances, with adequate, liberal ointment application, discomfort is kept to a minimum.

Prescription pain medication may be needed for the first one or two days.

Specific Risks

❖ Milia (cysts that look like whiteheads) may form in the treated area.

❖ Hypertrophic or keloid scar formation is a common risk in patients who have deep dermabrasion. For this reason, multiple superficial treatments are preferable to a single deep abrasion.

❖ Permanent pigment changes, especially bleaching, are possible with deep dermabrasion.

❖ During initial healing, the skin must be protected against infection. Take care to wash your hands thoroughly before touching your face. Do not pick or scratch the treated area. *If you experience itching, it is due to dryness in the treated area. Apply ointment more frequently or more liberally to reduce the discomfort.*

❖ If itching persists in spite of additional use of ointment, you may be sensitive to the ointment itself. Consult your doctor, as you may need to change medications.

❖ Pigmentation changes may become permanent if skin is exposed to the sun soon after the operation.

Recovery Time

Return to Work:
You can return to work within two or three days if you are working indoors. Patients who have had extensive facial dermabrasion will require a week to ten days of recuperation before returning to work.

If you have a job that may expose your freshly treated skin to environmental hazards (sun, extremes in temperature, soot and airborne pollutants, etc.) consult your physician before returning to work.

Exercise
There are no restrictions. Proceed with exercise as comfort allows, usually after four or five days.

Sex
Same as for exercise.

Sun
Stay out of the sun. Always use a sunscreen.

Travel
There are no restrictions on travel.

Frequency/Duration of Results

Depending upon your condition, multiple sessions spaced several months apart may be indicated. Results are permanent.

What to Expect

For the first few days, you will have oozing of plasma in the treated area. This will be unsightly if not managed properly; therefore, it is important to follow your doctor's instructions regarding cleansing and the application of medicated ointment.

The treated area will remain pink for several weeks or even months after treatment.

Extremes in temperature will aggravate the color of the treated area for several weeks or even months.

You may use corrective makeup once the crust separates.

Family members, especially small children, should be prepared for your postprocedure appearance.

You will need to use a sunblock.

Fees/Insurance

The cost of dermabrasion varies according to how much is being done, with an average price of $1,500 per treatment of each site.

The procedure may be covered by insurance if performed as a part of a medically indicated procedure. Get preapproval from your insurance carrier. Your doctor will advise you of conditions that may qualify for coverage.

Important Questions to Ask About Dermabrasion

❖ Will I need more than one treatment?

❖ What will the skin in the treated area look like?

❖ Do you use bandages?

❖ What do you recommend to camouflage my face as it is healing?

❖ What is a realistic recovery timetable for me?

Chemical Peel

Overview

It's hard for anyone to conceive of someone intentionally asking a doctor to put a strong caustic substance on their skin in the name of beauty. Many people do, often with dramatic results.

Most patients who seek out this procedure are experiencing the ravages of time, not to mention the self-inflicted abuses of sun exposure, smoking, and alcohol use. Telltale blotches and wrinkles are most commonly associated with the face and neck, but the observant critic will often look first at the hands.

Elizabeth is a vibrant fifty-eight-year-old grandmother. She was happy with her face and body, acknowledging that she looked well for any age. One of her joys was jewelry; however, she had stopped wearing some of her favorite pieces lest she draw attention to her "alligator hands" (her words, not mine). Brown spots and dry patches that refused to respond to even the most expensive lotions were the result of years on the golf course and in the garden.

A TCA peel accomplished two things: First, the unsightly brown patches were all lightened and, second, the

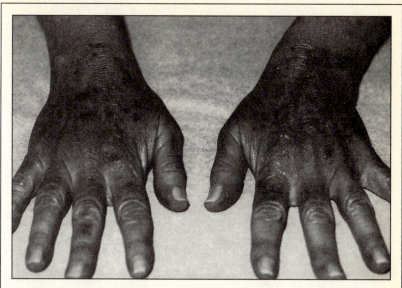

Chemical Peel of the Hands: Before, above, and a month after a TCA peel, below. The skin is still pink but the brown blotches and spots are already considerably lighter.

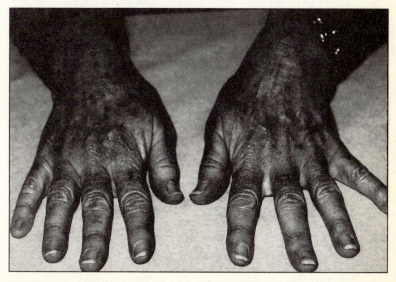

dry, crepey hide was replaced with thicker, smoother, healthier-looking skin. Elizabeth is wearing more jewelry today . . . and her husband has yet to forgive me.

Three Categories of Chemical Peels

There are three main categories of chemical peel, which explains the great variation in the description and experience with chemical peels from patient to patient.

For simplicity's sake, think of them as **weak** (alphahydroxy acids), **moderate** (trichloroacetic acid), and **strong** (phenol).

Alphahydroxy Acids (AHA)

Uses

❖ Good exfoliant that smooths rough, dry skin

❖ Improves texture of sun-damaged skin

❖ Can be used on skin of face and body

❖ Available in nonprescription strength in various cosmetics and salon facial treatments

❖ May be mixed with facial wash or cream in dilute concentrations as part of daily skin care regimen

❖ Can be mixed with bleaching agent to correct irregular pigmentation

❖ Aids in control of acne

❖ May be used as TCA pretreatment

What to Expect

❖ Multiple treatments (three to ten) are usually needed to achieve and maintain results

❖ Sessions usually spaced one to two weeks apart

- Nonprescription products may prolong results
- Treatment takes ten to fifteen minutes per session
- Use of sunblock recommended

Trichloroacetic Acid (TCA)

Uses
- Good exfoliant that smooths rough, dry skin
- Improves texture of sun-damaged skin
- Removes precancerous growths; *not to be considered treatment for skin cancer*
- Can be used on skin of face and body
- Smooths out fine to moderate surface wrinkles
- Lightens superficial pigmented blemishes
- Improves color and contour of some scars
- Useful in treating patients of all skin types, including African-Americans
- Often performed as adjunct to other plastic surgery procedures, e.g., face-lift

What to Expect
- May require pretreatment with AHA creams or Retin-A
- Depth of peel can be tailored to individual's skin
- Preferred for patients with darker skin
- Treatment takes thirty to forty-five minutes per session
- Requires frequent application of moisturizing ointment for first seven to ten days
- Healing is similar to recovering from a mild sunburn (without the pain) in seven to ten days

- Repeated treatment may be indicated to achieve desired results
- Two-month intervals between treatments recommended
- Use of sunblock required

Phenol

Uses
- Corrects coarse textural damage caused by sun, tobacco, alcohol, and medications (including oral contraceptives)
- Improves deep, coarse wrinkles
- Removes precancerous growths; *not to be considered treatment for skin cancer*
- Particularly useful in treating lipstick "bleed" lines
- May permanently remove freckles
- Often performed as adjunct to other plastic surgery procedures, i.e., face-lift

What to Expect
- A one-time procedure for most patients
- May only be used on face
- Requires heart monitoring during administration
- Not recommended for dark-skinned patients
- Full-face treatment will take one to two hours
- Recovery involves ten-day period of crusting followed by several weeks of redness requiring camouflage
- Sunblock must always be used
- Family, and especially small children, need to be prepared for your postpeel appearance
- Results are dramatic

The Procedure

Step 1: Pretreatment
There is usually no pretreatment for an AHA peel.

For a TCA or phenol peel, the skin is often pretreated with Retin-A for a period of one to two weeks.

Step 2: Preparation
All makeup use is stopped twenty-four to forty-eight hours before the procedure.

The skin is thoroughly cleansed of all makeup, lotions, perfumes, and skin oils immediately prior to the procedure.

Step 3: Degreasing
Using a substance such as acetone or alcohol, all remaining skin oils are removed.

Step 4: Anesthesia
For AHA, no anesthetic is required.

For TCA, no anesthetic is required for the lower concentrations. Sedation may be needed when higher concentrations are used.

For phenol, except for treating a very small area, sedation is needed as well as cardiac monitoring.

Step 5: Application
The AHA peel is usually applied with a soft fabric wipe.

TCA is applied, using swabs, wipes, or as a mist.

Phenol is applied slowly, in segments, using swabs. Because phenol can be absorbed systemically and is potentially toxic to the heart, it must be applied slowly and with careful cardiac monitoring.

Step 6: Dressing and Immediate Aftercare
AHA is self-limiting and usually does not need to be neutralized. If need be, it may be reversed by dilution with cool saline solution. This is seldom necessary. No dressing is

used. Makeup use is usually avoided for three hours. A moisturizing base containing a sunscreen is recommended before any makeup application. No other care is required.

After a TCA peel, the skin is treated with an antibiotic moisturizing ointment. This is needed for the first several days until the skin peels, much like after a sunburn. Makeup should not be worn until this process is completed. At that time, a moisturizing base containing a sunscreen is recommended with or without makeup.

After a phenol peel, the area is frequently covered with waterproof surgical tape. This helps to increase the depth and uniformity of the peel. Once the dressing is removed, petroleum jelly or a similar substance is used to moisturize your healing skin. This process takes seven to ten days.

Step 7: Recovery and Maintenance
There is no significant recovery period after an AHA peel. It is important to keep the skin moisturized and protected by a sunblock. You will notice some increased sensitivity to extremes of temperature. Common sense precautions are all that are required. Three to ten treatments spaced a week or two apart are generally required to achieve desired results. The process is repeated when necessary.

TCA recovery requires conscientious sunscreen protection and moisturizing. You may need to use camouflage makeup for two to three weeks, until any blotches of pink resolve. The procedure may be repeated any time after two months. It is unlikely that more than three TCA treatments will be performed in a single cycle. A maintenance peel might be recommended after one and a half to two years. Retin-A use will extend the period between treatments.

Recovery from a phenol peel often requires use of prescription pain medication and a significant recuperation time. After the crust separates at seven to ten days, a period of several months may be required for resolution of postprocedure redness. Expect that you will be very sensitive to extremes of temperature for the first year. Sunblock must become a daily part of your skin care routine.

In/Outpatient

Peels are done as outpatient procedures, usually in a doctor's office. For those requiring sedation and/or cardiac monitoring, an ambulatory surgical facility is required.

Incisions/Scarring

There are no incisions for chemical peels.

There is no significant risk of scarring in AHA peels and minimal risk in TCA peels.

Hypertrophic scars and keloid formation are recognized complications of deep phenol peels. These occur most often in the neck region. For this reason, application of phenol peels to the neck is not recommended.

Pain

For an AHA peel, mild to moderate stinging is common for up to three minutes. There is no other discomfort. Pain medication is not prescribed.

A TCA peel is similar to the application of a strong sports cream or liniment. There is a sensation of intense heat for three to five minutes. (It may seem longer, but it's not.) Then you will feel a dryness similar to that felt after application of a facial mask. This sensation is relieved once the antibacterial ointment is applied. There is no subsequent discomfort, even though you look like you have a sunburn.

Phenol peels hurt, and you may require prescription pain medication for the first few days, depending upon the size of the area being treated. Remember, you will be sensitive to extremes of temperature (pain medication won't help that) so you must take appropriate precautions.

Specific Risks

- Hypertrophic scar and keloid formation are possible complications with high concentrations of TCA and phenol.

- Permanent depigmentation (bleaching) is a risk, particularly in patients with dark complexions, with phenol. This does not mean that dark-skinned people cannot have peels, but they only need AHA or TCA.

- Cardiac dysrhythmias may be caused by phenol toxicity.

- Some degree of hypersensitivity to extremes of temperature is expected with all peels and is most significant with the higher concentrations of TCA and phenol.

Recovery Time

Return to Work
You can return to work immediately after an AHA peel.

After a TCA peel, you can return to work immediately, but you will look like you are sunburned for at least a week.

After a phenol peel, you will probably be able to return to work after ten days.

Exercise
There is no restriction to exercise after an AHA or TCA peel. Proceed as comfort allows after a phenol peel, usually after four or five days.

Sex
Same as for exercise.

Sun
Stay out of the sun. Always use a sunscreen. You will notice an increased sensitivity to the sun for at least a year after most peels.

Travel

There are no restrictions on travel.

Frequency/Duration

For AHA peel, usually three to ten treatments are spaced weekly or biweekly, for optimum results.

For TCA peel, one to three treatments are spaced at least two months apart to give optimum results.

A phenol peel is usually done in one session.

Results from any chemical peel process are positively affected by effective skin care, including use of substances such as Retin-A and suncreen. Adverse effects follow continuance of smoking, excessive alcohol consumption, and unprotected exposure to the sun. Some AHA protocols suggest monthly maintenance peels after the initial series of treatments. You may consider repeating a TCA peel in one to two years. Phenol peels are not generally repeated.

Fees/Insurance

The usual cost of chemical peels varies not only with the type of peeling agent used but also with the location and amount of work that is done. For example, TCA peel costs range from $1,200 to $1,500 for full face; $1,800 to $2,100 for chest, back, or hands and arms. Hands only will cost between $1,000 and $1,200. AHA peels cost between $60 and $100 per treatment, with three to ten treatments required for optimal results. Cost of phenol peels begins at at $750 for the area around the mouth and may be as high as $1,500 or $2,000.

This procedure is not usually covered by insurance unless it is used to treat a recognized medical condition. Be sure to get preapproval from your insurance carrier. Your doctor will advise you of any conditions that may justify coverage.

Important Questions to Ask About a Chemical Peel

❖ What type of peel is best for me?

❖ Will I need more than one treatment?

❖ What will the skin in the treated area look like? *(Ask for the worst-case scenario, not the best.)*

❖ How long will it look that way?

❖ What is a realistic recovery timetable for me?

Scar Revision Techniques

Overview

One of the most frequent and challenging demands placed on a plastic surgeon is the improvement of a scar. There is a pervasive misconception that plastic surgeons can remove scars, that is, restore the patient to their preinjured state. Would that it were true. A scar can never be completely erased, but it can usually be improved.

Scar revision techniques may mean making the scar less visible to the eye. They also frequently give the patient more flexibility and mobility in the damaged area.

There are few things more significant than a trauma that leaves daily reminders in the form of scars. It is understandable that patients and, indeed, physicians, want to intervene quickly after a scarring injury occurs. This is not always the wisest course to take because time is a great healer. Often, one of the most difficult things for surgeon and patient to do is nothing. The appearance of a mature scar is often much better than that of a fresh or immature scar. Scars may result from an automobile accident, a fall from a swing, a burn, an act of violence, or even a life-saving surgical procedure.

Peter was a twenty-four-year-old stockbroker who took great pleasure not only in sports and fitness training but also in his appearance. Many of his friends thought he was model material, much to his delight.

One Saturday afternoon, while bicycling in Central Park, he struck a rut and was thrown and knocked unconscious. When he awoke in the emergency room, he was told that he had life-threatening internal bleeding, which required an emergency operation. The next day, he found a large bandage on his abdomen and was then informed that his spleen had been removed. Because of his excellent physical condition, he recovered without complications. He was, however, left with a twenty-inch scar that ran from his breastbone to his pubis.

His doctor, expecting his patient's undying gratitude, was not prepared for his expressions of despair over the "mutilation" of his body. Life, as Peter knew it, was over.

Peter became a hermit. He no longer felt comfortable with any activity that might expose his scarred body. Not only did he refuse to go to the beach, he also would not go to the gym as he would have to disrobe in the shower.

A year later, when he came to me, he had a hypertrophic scar with characteristic "railroad track" scarring left from the heavy retention sutures that had been required in his emergency operation.

It took three preoperative visits to discuss realistic goals and expectations for scar revision. One of the most difficult things for Peter to accept was that there was no magic wand to make the scar vanish.

Once I was satisfied that his expectations were realistic, a series of two scar revision procedures were performed. The resulting scar was thinner and, though still obvious, much less conspicuous. Through the scar revisions and psychotherapy (a commonly recommended adjunct in severely traumatized patients) Peter has been able to return to the gym and a full, active life. His life priorities have been appropriately adjusted.

The Procedure

Every scar revision must be tailored to the individual. A common desire is to treat the entire scar at one time. For large scars, this is not recommended. Instead, a series of intermediary revisions tends to give more predictable—and satisfactory—results. There is nothing more frustrating than a failed scar revision.

The two most common complaints about scars are irregularities of contour—whether the scar is depressed or raised, wide or thick—and irregularities of color—whether it contrasts significantly with surrounding skin.

Depressed Scars

Depressed scars are often characterized by widening due to insufficient tissue. Revision frequently involves advancing healthy skin over the depressed area and securing it with fine sutures.

Raised Scars

With this type of scarring there is *too much* tissue. Revision involves resecting the excess scar tissue and advancing healthy skin in its place. Raised scars may also be treated with serial chemical peels or serial dermabrasion/dermaplaning.

Thick Scars

Keloid scars comprise the bulk of this category. Initial treatment of any thick scar usually involves injections of medications containing steroids to soften and flatten the scar while stopping production of additional scar tissue. This may be combined, particularly in burn patients, with an external compression dressing or garment that mechanically flattens the scar. As a last option, scar excision is undertaken. There is, however, a high rate of recurrence when excision is used to treat keloid scars, even when combined with irradiation therapy.

Color/Pigment Irregularities
Bleaching medications and chemical peels are frequently used to lighten dark or discolored scars. Surgical tattooing may be used to darken light scars.

Length of Procedure

Most serial scar revisions take less than an hour.

Anesthesia

Local anesthesia is commonly used, with or without the addition of sedation in most aspects of scar revision.

In/Outpatient

Most scar revision procedures are performed as an outpatient procedure.

Incisions/Scarring

Simple scar revisions follow the direct orientation of the scar being treated. When it is desirable to change the direction of the scar, a surgical technique such as a Z-plasty or W-plasty will be used. (See illustrations, page 174.)

Because plastic surgery is not an exact science, scar revision will result in a new scar that looks better, worse, or the same as when you started. This is a reason to begin with small steps.

Pain

Pain is not usually a significant factor in scar revisions.

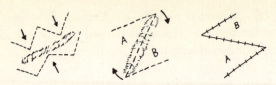

Scar Revision: While simple scar revision follows the orientation of the scar, more complex scars may require redirection. Left, W-plasty, in which the surgeon makes a W-shaped incision over the scar. Center, Z-plasty, calls for a Z-shaped incision through the scar. The two triangular-shaped flaps of skin, A and B, are transposed to reverse the direction of the scar (forming a backward Z), as shown on right. Existing scar tissue is excised and a new, less obvious albeit longer scar remains.

Specific Risks

✦ If your goals are unrealistic, you will not only be disappointed, but you will also be further emotionally traumatized by the scar revision.

✦ The scar may be made worse.

✦ In the case of keloids, a high incidence of recurrence can be expected.

✦ Pigmentation changes may become permanent if the scar is exposed to the sun soon after the operation.

✦ An immature scar may widen if stressed. It does you no good to have a scar revision and resume strenuous activity before the scar is mature (six weeks).

Recovery Time

Return to Work
✦ Desk job: Consult your doctor.
✦ Manual labor: Bending, lifting heavy weights, or straining are restricted. Your doctor will advise you as to when you can resume these activities.

Exercise
Don't do anything until you have worked out a program with your doctor.

Sex
Your doctor will advise you.

Sun
Stay out of the sun. Always use a sunscreen.

Travel
As a rule, there are no restrictions on travel by automobile, airplane, or bus.

Frequency/Duration of Results

Results are varied. Almost all scars improve with time.

What to Expect

You will still have a scar after any of the above procedures. While the goal is to make it as inconspicuous as possible, it will never be completely eliminated. *Beware of doctors who promise total elimination of a scar. If it sounds too good to be true, it probably is.*

For all but the smallest scars, a series of revisions is often the most appropriate course of treatment.

In all scar revisions, a new scar is formed, which takes just as long to mature as the original. Expect the same type of color changes, etc.

Because it takes a scar about forty-two days to mature (gain its full strength), a tape dressing is frequently applied to support the scar and minimize widening. This is left on for six weeks. If the scar is on the arm or leg, a cast or splint may be used for six weeks.

Expect your scar to improve slowly over a year.

Some procedures, such as W-plasty and Z-plasty, actually lengthen a scar in order to change the direction and improve the appearance of the scar.

For scars in general and keloids in particular, there are often multiple approaches. No one way is necessarily right or wrong. Discuss all options with your plastic surgeon.

Fees/Insurance

Cost of scar revision is determined by the type of procedure involved and the amount of work necessary.

Insurance coverage varies, depending upon the cause of the injury. For example, scars resulting from a motor vehicle accident are more likely to be covered than scarring caused by severe acne. Today, insurers insist that there be a *functional* component to scars (pain, limitation of motion, etc.) before reimbursing patients for scar revision.

Important Questions to Ask About Scar Revision

- ❖ Will I need more than one treatment?

- ❖ What will the skin in the treated area look like?

- ❖ Will I need an immobilizer (cast or splint)?

- ❖ What is a realistic recovery timetable for me?

- ❖ How can I camouflage the area being treated?

Sclerotherapy for Spider Vein Removal

Overview

Spider veins, also known as telangiectasias or sunburst varicosities, are tiny, nonessential veins that lie close to the surface of the skin. This condition occurs most often in women.

Unlike varicose veins, which are larger, darker in color, and more likely to bulge, spider veins are of little if any medical consequence. Varicose veins may cause pain and can be related to more serious vein disorders, which frequently require surgical treatment. Spider veins, on the other hand, can be injected with a solution that causes them to collapse and, in time, fade from view.

Heredity may play a part in this condition, as does pregnancy, hormonal shifts, weight gain, and certain medications. Occupations and activities that require prolonged sitting or standing may also be factors.

Two or more sclerotherapy sessions—performed at least one month apart—are required to achieve optimum results.

Serious medical complications from this purely cosmetic procedure are rare; however, sclerotherapy is not without risks. These include blood clots in the veins, allergic reactions to the sclerosing solution, inflammation, and skin injury that could result in permanent scarring.

In this procedure, which takes from fifteen to forty-five minutes per session, one injection is administered for every inch of spider vein—from five to forty per session. A cotton ball is secured with compression tape to each area of the leg as it is finished.

In addition to the compression tape applied during the procedure, you will wear tight-fitting support stockings to guard against blood clots and promote healing. After forty-eight hours, the cotton balls and tape can be removed; however, stockings should be worn for seventy-two hours or longer. You will be encouraged to walk to prevent clots from forming in the major veins, but during the time you are being treated, you should avoid prolonged periods of sitting or standing, as well as squatting, heavy lifting and extended running and jogging.

Sclerotherapy should not be considered a quick fix for spider veins. While bruising and redness at the injection sites will usually diminish within four to six weeks, pigmentation irregularities—brown splotches that look like tea stains—may take months, *sometimes as long as a year,* to fade. Additionally, new telangiectasias can develop at the margins of the treated areas, which, themselves, may require treatment.

Tattoo Removal

Overview

There are few things one regrets more than having had an ill-placed or ill-conceived tattoo. Frequently, these are permanent reminders of fleeting passions.

Tattoos may be classified as traumatic, amateur, or professional:

Traumatic tattooing is the result of an abrasion-type injury, such as skinning your knee on the sidewalk. In this case, some of the dirt and debris becomes incorporated into the wound as it heals, leaving a pigmented reminder of the injury.

Amateur tattooing, as the name suggests, are tattoos done by nonprofessionals. The pigment is placed very deeply and irregularly into the skin, usually using crude instruments.

Professional tattoos are those done by tattoo artists of varying talent and skill.

Tattoos are permanent because the pigment is ingested by specialized cells in the skin. Since the pigment is inert, it cannot be digested, and it remains a permanent part of the cell. Tattoo removal requires breaking up these cells to remove the pigment or totally removing the pigment-containing cells.

The first method of tattoo removal is excising, or cutting out, the offending area. This is obviously limited, depending upon the size and location of the tattoo.

A second method of tattoo removal is dermabrasion, discussed earlier in this chapter. This method is useful in traumatic tattoos, because the pigment is usually more superficially located. Professional tattoos also respond fairly well to this process, but amateur tattoos respond poorly because they are usually deeper. Multiple sessions are usually required to remove tattooing by the dermabrasion technique. One of the common side effects of this treatment is permanent bleaching of the surrounding skin.

A third method of tattoo removal employs laser technology, which is discussed in chapter 11 on pages 223–225.

Finally, certain tattoos, such as large or dark designs, are better camouflaged than removed. In such cases, over-tattooing is the treatment of choice. This should be done by someone experienced in surgical tattooing or a professional tattoo artist.

9

Hair Restoration

~

◆ **Male Pattern Baldness and Alopecia** ◆ **Transplants** ◆ **Flap Surgery** ◆ **Scalp Expansion** ◆ **Scalp Reduction**

Remember that *I Love Lucy* episode when Ricky was convinced he was losing his hair? Viewers got a big laugh out of Lucy's attempts to snap Ricky out of the dumps, especially when she piled a mountain of ugly gunk onto his head and massaged it into his scalp.

Baldness may be grist for the sit-com mill, but it is no laughing matter to the millions of men and women plagued by extensive hair loss. Yes, *women.* Experts estimate that one in five females experience some degree of severe hair loss.

We are supposed to lose *some* hair—between eighty and one hundred hairs per day—through attrition. This means that both the hair, with its root, and the scalp, with its complex network of nerves and glands, are working properly.

However, if you come out with a whole handful of hair when you run your fingers through it, or if you see a lot of hair on your pillow, in your brush or in the shower after washing, you have a problem. It could be that the *papilla,* or root, is dead, making new growth impossible.

How Hair Grows

Hair is dead—at least the part of it we see is. Only the bulblike papilla is alive, nourished by blood vessels throughout the scalp. Hair is 97 percent protein, with the remaining 3 percent composed of amino acids, minerals, and trace minerals.

A strand of hair or *follicle* grows about one-half inch per month for from two to six years, then it goes dormant for three to four months. During this respite, this hair is released by the papilla so that a new follicle can begin to grow. In time, the first strand is pushed out by the new hair that has been slowly making its way through the skin.

Under optimum conditions—when this growth-regrowth cycle is in working order—the average life span of a healthy human hair is four years.

As a rule, hair loss is primarily caused by a combination of aging, hormonal changes, and a family history of baldness. It also may be related to stress, illness, and medical treatment, including chemotherapy, radiation, and medications. Environmental conditions— intense pollution and airborne grit and grime—are extremely damaging to hair and scalp as well.

Male pattern baldness begins at the crown and/or temples and spreads. Degrees of baldness may range from receding hairlines to bald patches to almost complete hairlessness. I hesitate to use the term *premature* since just about any man who has lost his hair considers his balding to be premature, but premature balding may begin in the early to mid twenties.

Women most commonly experience thinning all over the scalp; however, patchy hair loss—*alopecia areata*—can also be a problem.

While balding is of little *physical* consequence, the emotional toll can be debilitating.

In all probability, a plastic surgeon won't be the first person you'll turn to, to take care of severe hair loss. No doubt you'll start with your barber or hair stylist and try every hair and scalp treatment you can find.

Inevitably, you'll see your family doctor or a dermatologist. You'll experiment with holistic and prescription medications, both topical and oral; vitamins, minerals, and other nutritional supplements; massage and perhaps even electrical stimulation, taking exceptional measures to avoid balding.

If you are considering taking the route of medications, consult a physician who has an extensive hair-replacement practice. Such products as minoxidil, commonly marketed as Rogaine™, may now be purchased without prescription, but I recommend that you exercise care and seek professional counseling before trying any medically based hair growth treatment. *Be aware that hair restored by medication falls out once you quit taking that medication.*

For some people, hair substitutes may provide a viable solution to moderate hair loss. This includes weaves, extensions, toupees, hair pieces, and full wigs. For others, nothing will do but for their scalp to be covered with live, *growing* hair. *That's* where plastic surgery can prove helpful. Just be aware that surgical hair transplants are not for everyone. What hair you have must be healthy and in enough quantity to survive the transplant process.

Overview

Candidates for surgical hair replacement must have healthy hair growth at the back and sides of the head to serve as donor areas for grafts and flaps. Other factors affecting the cosmetic result are hair color, texture, and amount of curl. Patients with dark, coarse hair will have more dense growth than those with fine or light-colored hair.

Hair replacement operations *can* be helpful in restoring a full—or fuller—head of hair; however, results won't necessarily match your dream.

Because of the sensitive issues of self-image, patients who seek this procedure need to find a surgeon who is not only clinically competent in the complexities of the process but is especially sympathetic to the emotional needs involved. Procedures are tedious, and results are not immediate—it takes 102 days for transplanted hair to grow.

Definitions

Graft   Living tissue is moved from one part of the body and put somewhere else. In general, round-shaped *punch grafts* usually contain ten to fifteen hairs. A *mini-graft* contains two to four hairs; a *micro-graft*, one to two. *Slit grafts*, which are inserted into slits created in the scalp, contain four to ten grafts each. *Strip grafts*, which are long and thin, contain thirty to forty hairs.

Flap transposition   This procedure involves lifting a flap of hair-bearing skin from the back of the head. While still attached at one end, the flap is rotated into position over the bald scalp. This procedure may be combined with scalp reduction.

Scalp expansion   The first stage of a two-stage procedure to bring hair together at the crown. A balloonlike tissue expander is inserted beneath the scalp and inflated in intervening weekly treatments over several weeks to stretch and loosen skin.

Scalp reduction   The second stage following scalp expansion and, on occasion, as part of flap transposition operations. The tissue expander is removed, and a segment of bald scalp is resected. The skin is brought together and sutured to cover the bald area.

The Procedure

For hair transplants, hair in the donor area will be trimmed so that grafts can be more easily harvested. The bald scalp is then cleaned with antiseptic. Grafts are then transplanted in a geometric pattern, usually along the front hairline, about one-eighth of an inch apart. Your surgeon will take care in removing and placing grafts so that the transplanted hair will grow in a natural direction and that hair growth in the donor site is not adversely affected. Donor site holes as well as transplanted areas will be closed with sutures.

Flap operations involve lifting a segment of hair-bearing skin from the back or side of the scalp, leaving it attached at one end. The flap is then rotated into the desired position, with the original blood supply undisturbed, and then sutured into place. Finally, the flap donor site is closed.

Tissue expansion is the first stage of a two-stage procedure to bring hair-bearing skin together at the crown. A balloonlike tissue expander is inserted through a small incision beneath the hair-bearing scalp and then inflated with a saline solution in intervening weekly treatments over several weeks to stretch the skin.

Tissue expansion is followed by scalp reduction. After removal of the expander, the segment of bald scalp is resected and hair-bearing skin is brought together. This reduces or eliminates the bald area.

Length of Procedure

Grafts: As a rule, several surgical sessions, lasting three to four hours per session, are needed to achieve satisfactory fullness. An average of 50 large plugs or 700 mini- or micrografts are transplanted at each session. With a healing interval of several months recommended between each session, this procedure may take up to two years to see full results.

Flap operations take less than two hours.

The initial stage of tissue expansion—insertion of the balloon—usually takes less than an hour. Over the next two to three months, weekly treatments involve inflation of the tissue expander, each taking about forty-five minutes.

Scalp reduction surgery takes less than two hours.

Anesthesia

You and your doctor have several options:

Local Anesthesia: Injection of anesthetic is used to numb the area being treated.

Local with Sedation: You will be put to sleep by medication administered into a vein, then local anesthesia with epinephrine will be injected into the area being treated.

General Anesthesia: You will be put to sleep, usually with gas, with a ventilator breathing for you.

Most hair replacement procedures, regardless of the technique, are performed under local anesthesia with sedation. General anesthesia may be used for more complex cases involving flaps, tissue expansion, or scalp reduction.

In/Outpatient

Most hair replacement procedures are performed in a surgeon's office or in an ambulatory surgery center as an outpatient.

Pain

As a rule, mild pain medication is prescribed for a week. Patients report varying degrees of aching, tightness, and throbbing.

Incisions/Scarring

The number of incisions and extent of scarring varies with the number and type of plugs and incisions. In general, scars are hidden by the hair.

Specific Risks

❖ Wide scars caused by tension may result from overzealous scalp-reduction procedures.

❖ Fluid or blood accumulation under the skin may resolve itself spontaneously or require surgical drainage.

❖ While it is normal for hair contained within the plugs to fall out before establishing regrowth in its new location, not all transplanted follicles survive to the extent that secondary procedures may be needed.

❖ Patients with large punch grafts may notice small bumps on the scalp at the donor or transplant site, like on a doll's head. For this reason, most opt for the smaller grafts (micro- and minigrafts).

❖ A patchy appearance occurs when newly placed hair lies next to patches of hair that continue to thin out. Should this happen, additional replacement procedures may be necessary.

Recovery Time

Return to Work
❖ Desk job: You can usually return to work within a week.
❖ Manual labor: Bending, lifting heavy weights, or straining are restricted for two to three weeks.

Exercise
Strenuous activity is restricted for at least three weeks after the operation.

Sex
Some doctors advise patients to avoid sexual activity for at least ten days after surgery. Don't try anything strenuous for a couple of weeks.

Sun
Stay out of the sun for the first week. Always wear a hat or scarf when out of doors.

Travel
There are no restrictions on travel by automobile, airplane, or bus.

Frequency/Duration of Results

For more natural-looking results, anticipate that you will need a touch-up procedure after your incisions have healed. This often involves blending, filling in the hairline with minigrafts, micrografts, or slit grafts. If you have a flap procedure, a small bump, or dog ear, may be visible on the scalp. This can be easily revised if it does not resolve itself spontaneously.

What to Expect

Surgical hair replacement will *not* turn back the clock and restore that full, youthful head of hair.

Expect that you won't see hair growth for months. It takes 102 days for a hair follicle to begin growth.

Expect some kind of head bandage that usually stays on for several days.

You may gently wash your head within two to three days following surgery.

Any sutures will be removed in a week to ten days.

Newly transplanted hair will fall out within six weeks after surgery. This condition is almost always temporary. It will take another five to six weeks before regrowth resumes.

A surgical touch-up is generally required to create a more natural-looking hairline.

A revision may be needed to eliminate a small dog-ear bump following flap or scalp reduction procedures.

Fees/Insurance

The cost of hair replacement surgery is determined by the procedure. You should know that some people charge by the plug. Because of variations in procedures—size of plugs or grafts, area of scalp affected, etc.—surgical fees vary greatly. This procedure is not usually covered by insurance.

Important Questions to Ask About Hair Replacement

❖ How many scars will there be, and will I be able to see them?

❖ Where will the scars be located?

❖ What will the treated area look like?

❖ What is the dressing like?

❖ What kind of special care will be required? (This may include ointments, special shampoos, special brushes, etc.)

❖ What is a realistic recovery timetable for me?

❖ What will I look like during my recovery time?

10

Just for Men

~

✦ Gynecomastia Correction ✦ Genital Procedures

The percentage of male plastic surgery patients has been on a steady rise since statistics were first compiled. As their numbers increased, so did their individual demands on the specialty to address problems unique to the male body.

Nearly every procedure described in this book can be applied to either a man or a woman. However, in this chapter, we will discuss procedures that are specific to males. These include correction of gynecomastia and reconstructive procedures relating to the form and function of the male genitalia. Usually, these latter procedures are performed by a team made up of the plastic surgeon, urologic surgeon, vascular surgeon and, when appropriate, pediatric surgeon.

Gynecomastia Correction (Male Breast Reduction)

Because men have such small amounts of breast tissue, most of us rarely give a man's *breasts* a thought—unless there is something wrong, as in the case of gynecomastia or male breast enlargement.

Breasts—female *or* male—are primarily composed of fat and glandular tissue, the development of which is governed by hormones. Sometimes this development goes awry.

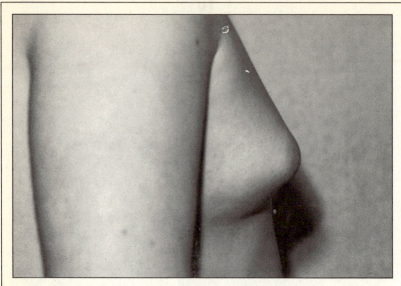

Gynecomastia Correction: Before, top, and three months after correction, bottom. Liposuction through small incisions at the bottom of each areola was used to aspirate breast tissue in this 15-year-old patient.

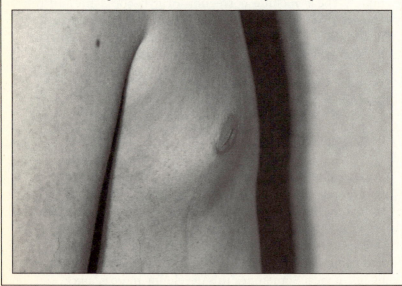

Vincent was a fifteen-year-old high school sophomore when his mom brought him to me. Through his sympathetic pediatrician, he had been diagnosed as having gynecomastia and was given a note excusing him indefinitely from participating in all phys. ed. activity. His breasts were the size of a woman's small B cup.

Vincent's mother, a single parent, while supportive, was most concerned because her son was becoming withdrawn, no longer participating in school activities. Even in summertime, he always wore heavy, baggy shirts to hide his condition.

Vincent's surgery was performed during summer vacation. His recovery was uneventful. It was not until he returned to school that the scope of his transformation became evident. Vincent tried out for the football team and, he proudly told me, he made the team, despite the fact that he had been excused from phys. ed. all those years. His renewed confidence was also reflected in his improved academic performance.

Serge, a twenty-six-year-old personal trainer when we met, had turned to body building and anabolic steroids in hopes that, if he had a big enough chest, no one would notice his breasts. In a way, this worked—provided he was fully clothed. At the gym, he always wore a workout uniform, including a tightly fitting undershirt, but he could never go shirtless because you would see the projection of his nipples.

Serge's operation and recuperation were successful, but three or four months later, he came in to say that his breasts were growing back. This had never happened to a patient of mine, and I was most perplexed.

Serge assured me that there was nothing else going on. As we were preparing to redo the operation, I pressed him as to whether or not he was using steroids again.

Finally, he admitted, "Well, not much." During his initial recuperation, he had started taking anabolic steroids to bulk up. Residual breast tissues had started growing again.

This condition required a second operation and now, almost five years later, Serge is doing fine. Serge is still a personal trainer, but he now concentrates more on aerobic activities than building mass.

Overview

From the Greek words for *womanlike breasts,* gynecomastia is a condition affecting an estimated 40 to 60 percent of men. This is *not* the breast associated with obesity. Instead, gynecomastia, which can affect one or both breasts, looks like the breasts of a female.

Gynecomastia often develops at puberty in 40 to 60 percent of young men when hormones are surging. However, 90 percent of all cases resolve themselves in a year or two. If this does not happen, the condition is considered permanent. Fortunately, it is correctable by plastic surgery. In the majority of cases, there is no identifiable cause for either the condition or its spontaneous resolution.

When gynecomastia develops later in life, it may be caused by a medical condition, such as impaired liver function or growth of a hormone-producing tumor. If this is the case, the first step is to identify and treat this medical problem. This may halt the progression of breast development but does not reduce the existing breast size.

Another source of this condition may be alcohol abuse or use of certain drugs, including anabolic steroids, estrogen-containing medications, and marijuana. Again, altering medications and stopping alcohol and drug abuse will halt the progression but frequently does not reverse the condition. Even after surgical correction, persistent use and abuse of these substances can cause the condition to return.

Excessive breast development can be psychologically debilitating at any age, but especially in the teen years, when body image is so important to one's identity. It is a challenge for parents to be supportive and understanding of their sons, many of whom may try to hide this condition from them.

Gynecomastia may be the reason behind difficulty at school and antisocial behavior (not wanting to participate in sports or physical education, refusing to go on family holidays to the beach, etc.) and isolation. Another clue to body image problems in teens might be a boy's refusal to wear anything but baggy sweatshirts, regardless of the weather or the occasion.

When gynecomastia persists into adulthood, the psychologic scars are no less significant. The pattern of antisocial behavior, while modified, continues. There is still the reluctance to participate in any activity in which the chest would be exposed and clothing is used to disguise the condition.

Many of these men turn to body building in hopes of developing a physique that would make their breasts less obvious. In fact, this serves to make the condition more obvious because the pectoral muscle development throws the excess breast tissue into a more projected position. Compounding this, some are misguided into thinking that anabolic steroids will be useful in their muscle development only to find out that they aggravate the condition and foster further breast growth.

Definitions

Anabolic steroids   A family of drugs with properties known to build body tissues, most notably muscles. In high doses, these drugs are converted by the body into feminizing hormones, which accounts for breast development in males and a host of other side effects, including acne and liver damage.

Areola   The pigmented area around the nipple.

Canula   A small, hollow tube. In liposuction it is inserted under the skin through one or more tiny incisions near the area to be suctioned. Attached to a syringe or vacuum pressure unit, the canula is guided by the surgeon to aspirate unwanted breast tissue.

Gynecomastia   Male breast enlargement.

The Procedure

There are two basic approaches to gynecomastia correction. Which method is used depends upon the ratio of fat to glandular tissue.

When the breast is composed primarily of fat (the vast majority of cases) liposuction, described in chapter 1, is the procedure of choice. The chest is infiltrated with a dilute anesthetic solution that makes it easier to aspirate fat while minimizing postoperative discomfort. The canula is inserted through a small incision (3 to 6 mm) at the bottom of the areola. The surgeon guides the canula, which is attached to a suction device, to aspirate the breast tissue. This technique gives the best contour and reduces the likelihood of developing a saucer deformity (see page 196). A compression garment is applied. Drains are seldom used.

In the infrequent instances where the breast is composed largely of glandular tissue, direct excision is combined with the liposuction technique described above. Dense glandular tissue is not aspirated as easily as fat through a suction canula and needs to be removed using a scalpel or surgical electrocautery device. Before the development of liposuction, this technique ran the risk of creating the saucer deformity. Now, combining the two techniques reduces this likelihood. A compression garment is applied. Drains may be used when the amount of direct excision is extensive.

Length of Procedure

Correction of gynecomastia usually takes approximately an hour and a half to two hours.

Anesthesia

You and your doctor have options:

Local with Sedation: You will be put to sleep with medication administered by vein. A local anesthetic with epinephrine is then injected into the area being treated.

General Anesthesia: You will be put to sleep, usually with a gas anesthetic, with a ventilator assisting your breathing.

Regardless of the chosen anesthetic, your doctor will use local anesthesia with epinephrine to reduce bleeding during the operation and aid in controlling postoperative pain.

In/Outpatient

Gynecomastia is generally performed as an outpatient procedure.

Incisions/Scarring

Most commonly, the incision is placed in the lower half of the areola where it will usually heal in an inconspicuous manner. A tape dressing may be used for the first few weeks to minimize widening of the scar. *If you have chest hair, don't trim or shave it as the hair will help to camouflage the incision as it heals.*

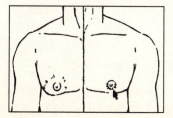

Gynecomastia Correction: Incisions are placed in the lower half of the areola (arrow) where they will heal in an inconspicuous manner. If additional excess skin must be removed, a larger incision may be required.

More extensive incisions are required if redundant or excess skin must be resected, but this is rarely necessary. If it is done at all, it is usually done as a second procedure.

Pain

You will feel very sore—achy muscle sore—much like you'd feel after a heavy workout. You will likely require prescription pain medication for up to a week, followed by over-the-counter medication for another week.

Specific Risks

- Skin loss, including loss of the nipple, is of concern primarily in patients who smoke. This may lead to significant scarring, which may require subsequent scar revision.

- Fluid or blood accumulation under the skin may resolve itself spontaneously or require a surgical drainage procedure.

- A craterlike contour irregularity described as a saucer deformity may develop if the margins of the resection are not feathered. This problem is largely avoided by using liposuction to remove the breast tissue.

- Asymmetry occurs frequently but is seldom permanent. If it persists, it can usually be corrected quite easily with a second limited procedure to smooth out the skin.

- Pigmentation changes, especially in the incision scar, may become permanent if the skin is exposed to the sun too soon after the operation.

Recovery Time

Return to Work
- Desk job: You can return to work as soon as you feel up to it—generally three or four days after the operation.

◆ Manual labor: Do not undertake bending, lifting heavy weights, or straining until you get your doctor's go-ahead. Avoid any activity that risks a blow to the chest area for at least four weeks.

Exercise

Moderate exercise is beneficial. You should begin walking as soon as comfort allows. Upper body exercises are restricted. Follow your doctor's recommendations.

Again, avoid all activity that risks a blow to the chest for at least four weeks.

Your doctor will tell you when you can resume weight training.

Sex

Take it easy for a week. Then, gradually increase activity with your doctor's guidance, taking special care to avoid any strenuous upper body activity.

Sun

Stay out of the sun for the first week. Always use sunscreen.

Travel

You may not feel like traveling for the first few days. After that, there are no restrictions to travel by automobile, airplane, or train. No bicycling for at least two weeks.

Frequency/Duration of Results

Results are permanent, but this does not mean you will be immune to the effects of substances known to cause breast growth. This is because it is impossible to remove all breast tissue and any remaining tissue will respond to substances such as anabolic steroids.

What to Expect

You will wake up from the operation in a compression vest, usually made out of elastic and Velcro®. You will wear the vest night and day, except when showering, for the first week to ten days. Depending upon the amount of excess skin, you may be instructed to continue wearing the compression vest or a skintight undershirt for an additional month to maximize skin contraction and minimize the likelihood of a second procedure for skin resection. *Bear this in mind when you schedule your operation because the vest can be uncomfortable in hot weather.*

You can expect a moderate amount of swelling and bruising, which will peak at three to four days and will resolve over the next month. Nipple sensation will be diminished following the operation and usually returns to normal within three months.

You will be instructed to restrict your arm movement, keeping your elbows to your sides for a week, followed by gradual increases in range of motion over the next two to three weeks. All weight-lifting activity will be restricted for up to six weeks (see the advice about exercise on page 197). Your doctor will develop a program with you.

Fees/Insurance

The usual cost of gynecomastia correction is between $3,500 and $4,500 for liposuction only. When resection of excess skin is required, this cost may be from $5,500 to $6,500.

This procedure is usually covered by insurance, but policies vary greatly. Check with your insurance carrier and get written preauthorization for any treatment recommended by your primary care physician. It is easier to get insurance reimbursement when the operation is performed in your teens. Once you are older, you may have more difficulty, but persistence usually pays off.

Important Questions to Ask About Gynecomastia Correction

❖ How many scars will there be?

❖ Where will they be? (Ask your surgeon to draw lines or dots with a marker where the incisions will be made.)

❖ What will the skin in the treated area look like?

❖ Will I have to have another operation to remove any excess skin?

❖ What is the compression vest like?

❖ Will drains be used?

❖ What is a realistic recovery timetable for me?

Cancer of the Male Breast

While there is no correlation between the presence of gynecomastia and the development of breast cancer in men, it is important to remember that 1 percent of all breast cancers occur in men. Men *can* get breast cancer. Have any suspicious lumps or changes in your nipples examined by your family physician.

Genital Procedures

Plastic surgeons are often called upon to play a role in the management of problems of male genitalia. These problems may be present at birth, in the form of congenital abnormalities such as hypospadias, or they may be acquired later in life through trauma or disease, resulting in tissue loss or impairment of function, such as impotency and inability to urinate.

❖ *Hypospadias:* This is a relatively common congenital anomaly in which the urethra does not extend to the end of the penis and opens elsewhere on the shaft. Correction is ideally performed in childhood but can be performed at any age. Repair is accomplished by a combination of flaps and grafts to obtain the best functional and cosmetic results.

❖ *Diseases and Traumatic Injuries to the Penis:* Surgical diseases of the penis usually result in a deformity that limits function. Correction is individualized but usually involves resection of diseased tissue and replacement with transferred tissue or prosthetic material. Traumatic injuries ranging from near total amputation to partial loss are reconstructed with any of a variety of local flaps or, more commonly, with microsurgical techniques.

❖ *Impotence:* Surgically correctable impotence that might be treated by the plastic surgeon is the consequence of such chronic diseases as diabetes and atherosclerosis. Patients with injuries that compromise the nerve supply to the penis may also be treated by the plastic surgeon.

In cases of blockage of the arteries that supply the penis, microsurgical arterial bypass or reconstruction is performed. In a similar fashion, traumatic injuries to the nerves supplying the penis may lend themselves to microsurgical repair. A variety of devices, ranging from penile implants to testicular prostheses, are used in cases where vascular or nerve repair is not possible.

In all cases of impotence, a major component of treatment involves pre- and postoperative psychologic counseling and support.

Penile Enhancement Procedures

There are two penile enhancement techniques currently gaining media attention, which are mentioned here with great reservation. They are performed on men with anatomically and functionally normal penises. The first is fat injection to enhance penis size, and the second is the so-called penis lengthening operation.

The injection of fat into the penis to increase its bulk is relatively new, unproven as safe, and unregulated. In this procedure, fat is harvested from another part of the body for injection beneath the skin of the penis.

Penis lengthening operations add nothing to the length of the penis. The procedure involves cutting the suspensory ligament of the penis at its attachment to the pubis. Advocates report that this adds up to one inch in "length" to the flaccid penis.

The American Society of Plastic and Reconstructive Surgeons strongly cautions patients considering using fat to augment the penis. As mentioned in chapter 11 on page 206, the success of fat injection for tissue enhancement varies greatly from individual to individual. It is not known why injected fat survives for extended periods of time in one patient and for only a short time in another.

Even if you are willing to accept the risk of failure of the fat graft, you are putting yourself at risk of very significant adverse effects, including but not limited to infection, skin loss, loss of sensation, and even loss of function.

With regard to the surgical "lengthening" of the penis, understand that the flaccid penis *appears* longer because its foundation and support has been severed. In addition to the risks of infection, skin loss, and sensory loss, there is a risk of functional compromise of the erect penis as a result of this loss of support.

Patients who are considering either of these cosmetic procedures are strongly encouraged to discuss their desires with a board-certified plastic surgeon who has specific training and expertise in this area. Psychologic evaluation to discuss motives and expectations may prove invaluable.

A final warning: There are no state or federal laws that mandate training and qualification for individuals who call themselves "medical specialists" and perform fat injection penile augmentation or penile lengthening procedures.

11

Reconstructive Procedures and Emerging Technologies

~

❖ Craniofacial Procedures ❖ Injectable Fillers ❖ Implants ❖ Microsurgery ❖ Endoscopy ❖ Laser Plastic Surgery ❖ Ultrasound

Reconstructive plastic surgery is the spiritual heart of this medical specialty. In fact, it was an operation to repair a damaged hand that first attracted me to the field.

The greatest advances in reconstructive surgery were born of necessity in treating burns and other injuries, stemming from the World Wars, when surgeons sought to close wounds, repair injured limbs, and replace lost tissue. The lessons learned in treating these horrors of war were then applied to the correction of congenital defects and repair of abnormalities resulting from trauma or disease. These same principles were applied in developing the aesthetic procedures used in *cosmetic* surgery.

The primary goal of *all* plastic surgery is to improve or restore function. Frequently, this process results in an improvement in form. Reconstructive surgery is seldom purely functional or purely cosmetic. Things that work better generally look better.

It is impossible to discuss every reconstructive procedure, but we will discuss the cosmetic aspects of some reconstructive plastic surgery for adults.

We also discuss the advances in technology that are shaping plastic surgery as it prepares to enter the twenty-first century.

From the perspective of recent history, the control of pain and the treatment of infection through developments in anesthesia and pharmacology have made it possible for physicians and surgeons to treat the injured and burned in ways never before possible. Instead of requiring amputation, a limb may be salvaged, and the patient with serious burns is less likely to succumb to overwhelming systemic infection.

Craniofacial Procedures

As a child, Mary was all arms and legs. As she grew into adulthood, her facial features began to change insidiously. Her eyes and eyelids began to bulge. She consulted her family doctor because of irregularities in her heartbeat. He also noticed changes in her skin and hair.

Mary was diagnosed as having Graves' disease (hyperthyroidism). She began treatment with medication and was cured of her disease. Although she was chemically normal, her eyes remained unchanged.

Mary was in her early thirties when she came to me to see if there was anything that could be done. Her problem, common to patients who have had Graves' disease, was that there was too much tissue to fit into the orbit or eye socket. Unlike other areas in the body where excess tissue is expendable, the eyeball and its surrounding musculature are vital.

The solution to Mary's problem was the enlargement of the orbit, or eye socket. This approach was extrapolated from treatment of fractures of the orbit, commonly known as "blow-out" fractures. When the eye sustains a blow of sufficient force, the floor of the orbit breaks to absorb this force and leave the eyeball intact. As a result of the injury, the eyeball and its surrounding tissue retract within the socket.

A problem in one case—the blow-out fracture—becomes the solution in another—Mary's case.

Through a subcilliary incision, a portion of Mary's orbital wall was removed on each side. This enlarged the rigid confines of the eye socket, allowing the eyeball to retract.

Mary's recuperation was uneventful and, in a week, she returned to her secretarial job a new woman with a brighter outlook on life.

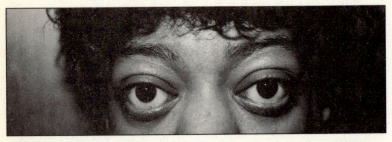

Repositioning of Eyes: Before, top, and after, bottom. The sockets were enlarged to accommodate the eyeballs and their surrounding muscle tissue through incisions placed under the eyelashes. The patient returned to work after a week, and six months after the operation had no obvious scars.

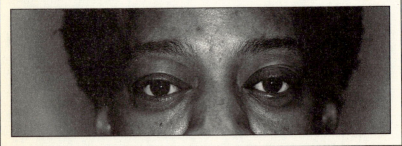

Overview

Craniofacial procedures involve resection and repositioning of segments of the skull and facial bones. Most of the operations result from our understanding and treatment of fractures of the skull and facial bones.

Frequently, as in the above-mentioned case study, a controlled fracture is made, excess bone is resected or deficient bone is replaced, and the pieces are held together with surgical wires, screws, or plates.

Patients who are candidates for craniofacial procedures are usually evaluated by an interdisciplinary team at medical centers that specialize in such care.

A large segment of craniofacial procedures involves treatment of the teeth and jaw. In these instances, the cooperation between plastic surgery and dental and orthodontic surgery is mandated. When segments of the skull are involved, a neurosurgeon is incorporated into the team.

It is not uncommon in major cases of craniofacial reconstruction for the team to include a plastic surgeon, neurosurgeon, orthodontist, oral surgeon, anesthesiologist, psychologist, and speech pathologist.

Emerging Technologies

As an outgrowth of the space program, our vocabulary has increased. Titanium, silicone, Teflon®, Gortex®, and other lightweight, durable materials, as well as fiber-optic cable, ultrasound, and laser technologies, have found their way into the medical arena. The same futuristic materials and technologies that sent a man to the moon are now being used to make precision surgical instruments. Some of these materials are even implanted to replace joints or augment missing tissue.

Injectable Fillers

Of historical note: Beginning in the late 1950s, liquid silicone was injected into breasts to enhance their shape and size. Significant and severe complications—specifically hardening of the breast, skin ulceration, and inability to differentiate silicone-related scar from breast cancer—resulted in an FDA ban on its use in this manner. Today, some advocate use of liquid silicone as a filler for facial wrinkles. Anyone receiving silicone injections for this purpose should be participating in an ongoing FDA-approved study.

Overview

Injectable fillers are used to improve facial skin texture. This can range from reduction of the depth of wrinkles or facial scars to enhancement of the lips or cheekbones. Frequently, fillers are used as adjuncts to other plastic surgery procedures or as temporizing steps to avoid or delay more extensive plastic surgery. The most common approved injectable fillers in use today are collagen and fat.

Collagen is the major protein of connective tissue that makes up the foundation of skin and other tissues. This treatment is not advisable for pregnant women, patients who are allergic to beef or bovine products, patients who suffer from autoimmune diseases, or those who are allergic to lidocaine, the local anesthetic mixed with the collagen.

Fat is adipose tissue from the patient's own body.

It is important to remember that while injectable fillers may provide a long-lasting improvement in the contour of the skin that is treated, they are not permanent solutions. Eventually, the body will metabolize or digest these substances and you will return to your original condition. There is no way to predict in advance how long your specific results will last. Repeat injections are required to maintain these effects.

When one injectable filler does not yield the desired long-lasting results, it is not to say that another will do the same. Be aware that *none* of them may work for you, either.

Fortunately, failure of injectable fillers to provide long-lasting results simply leaves you right where you started.

The Procedure

Because collagen for injection is an extract of animal skin, a skin test is required to make sure that you are not allergic to it. The skin test must be done one month before your first collagen treatment. Once your skin test is read as negative, you may begin treatment.

The injection is administered through a fine needle at several points along the treatment area. You will feel the injection, even though the material contains a local anesthetic.

Unlike collagen, when fat is used as the filler, it is taken from your own body. Consequently, there is no risk of allergic reaction. The donor site is anesthetized with a local anesthetic, the harvested fat is then "washed" to remove any impurities, and it is finally injected into the recipient site, which also has been anesthetized. Once the fat has been extracted and processed, it is injected in a similar manner as collagen.

Length of Procedure

Collagen injections require less than ten minutes per site.

Fat injections take less than thirty minutes. The most time-consuming part of this procedure is the harvesting of fat from the donor site.

Anesthesia

Collagen for injection contains local anesthetic.

Fat grafting requires use of local anesthetic in both the donor and recipient sites.

In/Outpatient

All procedures are usually done in the office, unless combined with another surgical procedure.

Incisions/Scarring

There are no incisions, and, unless there is an infection or serious allergic reaction, there should be no additional scarring.

Pain

You will definitely feel the injection. Local anesthesia reduces the discomfort, but some areas, such as the lips, are more sensitive than others, such as the cheeks.

Specific Risks

- The primary risk with collagen injection is allergic reaction either to the collagen itself or to the lidocaine anesthetic it contains. This may appear as redness, itching, or swelling at the injection site. This is rare but bears note. When it does occur, it is often aggravated by alcohol consumption.

- Infection, abscess, skin ulcers, skin loss, scarring, and lumpiness are *very* rare risks of collagen injections.

- With fat injections, there is a slight risk of lumpiness and a small risk of infection.

Recovery Time

Return to Work
There is usually no restriction on your return to work after receiving injectable fillers.

Exercise

Usually, there is no restriction on exercise after receiving injectable fillers. Check with your doctor first.

Sex

See exercise.

Sun

Stay out of the sun for the first week. Always use sunscreen.

Travel

There are no restrictions on travel by automobile, airplane, or bus.

Frequency/Duration of Results

Results are temporary, ranging from a few weeks to several months. Think of these procedures as applying a long-lasting makeup which, at some point, wears off and needs to be reapplied.

What to Expect

Because collagen injections contain some salt water, there will be minor swelling in the treated area for a day, until the body absorbs it.

Cold compresses applied immediately to each injection site will reduce swelling and the minimal redness that occurs after injection of any filler material. They will also reduce the chance of bruising.

With fat grafts, overcorrection is usually required because half of the fat injected will be resorbed within a week. This means that you will appear puffy or overdone during this time.

Remember: All injectable fillers are digested by the body and you will eventually return to where you started unless you have the procedure repeated.

Any lumpiness or asymmetry is self-limited and almost never requires correction.

Antibiotics are frequently prescribed prophylactically with fat injection.

Fees/Insurance

The usual cost of a collagen skin test is less than $100. Cost of injection of collagen is approximately $400 per syringe. A syringe contains 1 cc of collagen, which is an adequate volume to treat most cases.

Fat grafts begin at $750.

These procedures are not usually covered by insurance unless medically indicated, such as in treating a scar or indented area caused by an accident or injury.

Important Questions to Ask About Injectable Fillers

* What will the skin in the treated area look like?

* Will I have to wear a compression garment on the donor site for my fat graft?

* How much overcorrection or swelling should I expect? For how long?

* What is a realistic recovery timetable for me?

Implants

The development of silicone implants that can be easily molded gives rise to a variety of applications, from the enhancement of deficient facial structures—cheekbones, jaw, and chin—and filling out wrinkles and scars to contouring the chest, calf, and buttocks. Unlike injectable liquid fillers, these implants are semisolids.

Implants are not new to reconstructive plastic surgery, where they are used to restore lost facial tissue and to correct congenital and traumatic deformities. One rapidly growing area of cosmetic surgery involves augmentation of the chest, calf, and buttock areas with molded silicone implants. This field is generating much interest in the media but still is not widely embraced by all plastic surgeons.

Semisolid silicone implants are placed through incisions in the axilla for the chest, in the gluteal crease for the buttocks, and behind the knee for the calf. Implants are positioned deep to the muscles they seek to augment in the case of the buttocks and chest or beneath dense fascia for the calf.

In addition to patients with congenital defects, such as Poland's syndrome, in which a pectoral muscle is absent, and polio patients with atrophied muscles, those seeking body contouring implants include body-conscious men who, for whatever reasons, are unable to do the body work to develop and maintain a fit body, and body builders of both sexes who want to define specific areas of their bodies—usually the chest, buttocks, or calves.

Chest implants, positioned under the pectoral muscles, enhance the contour of the upper chest. While this initially was exclusively for men, female body builders who have diminished breast tissue mass as a result of their exercise programs may turn to chest implants to create the illusion of cleavage without the more obvious traditional breast implant.

In addition to adding definition, implants may be employed to camouflage depressions caused by torn muscles. A common injury for body builders, especially during bench press exercises, and athletes competing in high-impact sports, this generally involves a separation or tear of a portion of the pectoralis muscle. This often results in a bulging groove at the site of the tear. When surgical repair is not possible, the defect can be camouflaged by individually sculpted implants inserted through an axillary incision.

Early studies report modest success with sometimes very significant complications. The major complications are infection, collections of fluid or blood around the implant, rotation or displacement of the implants, or even extrusion of the implant.

Before undertaking any such procedure, discuss the various alternatives and risks with a qualified plastic surgeon who is experienced in this technique.

Overview

Implants range from pieces of your own soft tissue, such as fascia taken from your temple or thigh, to pieces of cartilage harvested from your nose or ear, to synthetic thread-like strips of materials such as Gortex®. Other synthetic implants are largely made up of semisolid silicone that has been shaped to the specific area to be enhanced. Finally, bone, taken from your hip or skull, may be implanted in more extensive facial reconstructive procedures.

Bone, fascia, and cartilage have the potential to be incorporated into the recipient area as living tissue. If this process fails, they may be partially or totally resorbed by the body.

Implants made of synthetic substances are usually biologically inert and therefore remain unchanged. However, the body may respond to the implanted material by forming a capsule or scar around the implant.

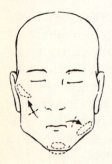

Facial Implants: Custom-shaped implants for the cheeks, jaw and chin are inserted through incisions in the mouth.

The Procedure

If bone, cartilage, or fascia are being used as implants, they must be harvested. The usual donor sites for bone are the hip and skull. The nose and ear are potential sources for cartilage grafts. Finally, the side of the thigh or temple provide fascia for grafting.

Strip grafts made of fascia or Gortex® are frequently used to fill out the nasolabial line or to augment the lips. Insertion requires use of a local anesthetic and involves threading the graft into place using a straight needle, similar to a sewing needle.

As a rule, synthetic facial implants are used to augment the cheeks, chin, nose, or jaw. Since each procedure is individualized to the specific patient, each implant must be individualized. Measurements are taken, preoperatively, and an appropriately sized implant is chosen.

Bone implants are used to reconstruct large segments of missing facial bone. This follows the precept in plastic surgery of replacing like tissue with like tissue whenever possible.

Chin Implants

Chin implants augment a weak chin, giving you a stronger, better-defined profile. An incision is made either inside the lower lip or in the crease under the chin. A small pocket is fashioned to hold the implant, which is slipped into position. After the incision is closed, a tape dressing is applied, much like the chin strap on a football helmet.

Cheek Implants

As the name suggests, these implants increase the definition of your cheekbones. When they are inserted in conjunction with another procedure, such as a face-lift or eyelid operation, the same incisions are used for implant placement. If cheek implants are placed by themselves, then an incision is placed inside the upper lip or on the lower eyelid. Through the incision, a pocket is fashioned to hold the implant in place on the cheekbone. A dressing may be used.

Lower Jaw Implants

The least-frequently performed facial implant procedure corrects deficiencies of the side of the jaw or jawline. An internal incision is made on either side of the lower lip and, again, pockets are fashioned to hold the implants in place. Dressings are not usually employed.

Nasal Implants

Nasal implants may be bone, cartilage, or synthetic. These are always placed in conjunction with rhinoplasty and are more frequently used to correct deformities resulting from previous operations or trauma. Implants are also used to modify hereditary traits, such as a broad or flat nose.

Chest Implants

Inserted through an axillary incision, chest implants are positioned above the nipple to fill out the upper chest. They provide definition to the upper pectoralis muscles or may be used to camouflage bulging grooves resulting from a tear in this muscle. Female competitive body builders who seek enhanced cleavage often opt for pectoral implants rather than traditional breast implants for a more natural look.

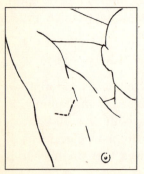

Chest Implants: Chest or pectoral implants are inserted through an incision placed in the axillary crease and positioned above the nipples to fill out the upper chest.

Buttocks Implants

Inserted under the gluteus maximus muscle through an incision in the midgluteal crease—just above the coccyx—semisolid silicone implants enhance the contour of the upper buttocks. This procedure may be combined with liposuction of the thighs and saddlebags.

Calf Implants

Used to correct underdeveloped or atrophied muscles, calf implantation is now being sought by athletes—especially body builders—to obtain a shape and volume that is impossible through exercise. Other candidates for calf implantation are women with poorly defined calf musculature. Implantation is often combined with liposuction of the knees and ankles.

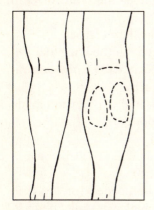

Calf Implants: Working through incisions in the fold behind the knees, implants are positioned on either or both sides of the calf as needed to enhance poorly defined calf musculature.

Length of Procedure

Chin implants take from thirty to sixty minutes to perform. Cheek implants require thirty to forty-five minutes. More complex, jaw and nasal implants require one to two hours.

Chest and buttocks implants take approximately one to one and a half hours and calf implants require thirty to forty-five minutes.

Anesthesia

Many facial implants can be placed using local anesthesia alone. It is common, however, to use local anesthesia with sedation. Complex procedures require use of a general anesthetic.

In/Outpatient

As a rule, implants are done as an outpatient procedure in an ambulatory surgery facility.

Incisions/Scarring

For facial implants, many incisions are placed intraorally. If external incisions are used, they are in the lower eyelid for cheek implants and in the crease under the chin for chin implants.

Chest incisions are placed in the axillary crease.

For calf implants, incisions are made in the knee fold. *Incisions must be taped for six weeks.* Scars will be obvious initially but usually heal quite satisfactorily.

Buttocks implants are inserted through an incision made in the buttock crease, above the tailbone.

Pain

Prescription pain medication will be needed for the first three to five days. Over-the-counter analgesics may be indicated for one to two weeks.

Severe pain may be indicative of problems.

Specific Risks

❖ Severe pain may be indicative of problems.

❖ Bleeding around an implant may cause a medical emergency known as compartment syndrome. This condition, if not treated immediately, results in pressure necrosis that cuts off circulation to muscles and nerves, causing them to atrophy and stop functioning.

❖ Fluid or blood accumulation around the implant may resolve itself spontaneously or require surgical drainage.

❖ Any infection around an implant will usually be treated with antibiotics. If an infection persists, then the implant itself may need to be removed and replaced in a second operation after the infection is resolved.

❖ An implant may become dislodged. Usually this is caused by trauma. If this occurs, a second operation may be required to reposition the implant.

❖ In some cases, pressure caused by the presence of the implant may erode underlying bone.

Recovery Time

Return to Work
❖ Desk job: Most people return to work within a week.
❖ Manual labor: Bending, lifting heavy weights, or straining are restricted for a month.

Avoid any activity that risks a blow to the face or the area where implants are positioned.

Exercise
Begin walking around as soon as comfort allows.

Do not resume *any* exercise program without your doctor's permission.

With chest implants, exercise, including weight lifting, is restricted for six weeks.

Sex
Your doctor may advise you to wait for a week or two.

Sun
Stay out of the sun. Always use sunscreen.

Travel
There are no restrictions on travel by automobile, airplane, or bus. You may not feel like taking an extended trip for about a week.

Frequency/Duration of Results

Results are usually permanent when semisolid silicone gel implants are used.

Bone, cartilage, or fascial implants may be resorbed by the body.

What to Expect

The area around any implant will be bruised and swollen for seven to ten days.

You will require prescription pain medication for three to five days.

Any intraoral incision requires special care. Your diet will be restricted, usually to soft, bland foods. Oral hygiene will be important. Be sure that you understand your doctor's protocol *completely* and follow it.

Intraoral sutures usually dissolve within ten days.

Antibiotics are usually prescribed as a prophylaxis for up to ten days.

Expect two black eyes after cheek implants. You may or may not get them. If you do, it takes a week to ten days for them to resolve.

You will need to keep your head elevated at all times, including at night, for the first week, as this will reduce bruising and swelling. *A recliner will keep you in the proper position.*

Cold compresses are generally applied at frequent intervals for the first twenty-four hours to minimize bruising and swelling. *Frozen peas in a zip-top plastic bag wrapped in a hand towel make an excellent compress.*

After twenty-four hours, you may find that warm compresses help to resolve bruising and swelling. *Some patients prefer to continue cold compresses during this time, but most find warm compresses beneficial.*

In calf implant operations, incisions must be taped for six weeks for optimal results.

Hydroquinone, a skin bleaching medication, is frequently prescribed to prevent or treat hyperpigmentation of the scars from calf implantation.

A compression bandage or garment is usually recommended for chest implants for the first one to two weeks.

Fees/Insurance

The usual cost of facial implants is between $750 and $2,500 per implant.

Pectoral implants cost approximately $2,500 to $3,500 per implant.

Buttocks implants range from $1,000 to $2,750.

Calf implants cost between $1,000 and $3,000.

These procedures are not usually covered by insurance unless performed as part of a medically indicated reconstruction.

Important Questions to Ask About Implants

❖ How many scars will there be?

❖ Where will they be?

❖ What will the skin in the treated area look like?

❖ What is the dressing like?

❖ Will I be on a special diet?

❖ Will any incisions in my mouth need special care?

❖ What is a realistic recovery timetable for me?

Microsurgery

Overview

Every student of science will remember the significance of the discovery of the microscope. The constant refinement of the optics of this instrument follow the development of diagnosis and treatment of diseases throughout modern history.

Beginning in the 1960s, with the experimental application of the microscope to the operating room—specifically in the field of neurosurgery—a new subspecialist, the microsurgeon, emerged. Refinements in optics, coupled with development of microsurgical instruments such as sutures many times finer than a human hair and the clamps precise enough to hold them, lead to the manufacture of affordable operating microscopes. Today, virtually every hospital operating arena offers this technology and microsurgical training is now a basic element of surgical education.

Today's surgeon performs operations that were previously thought impossible, whether it be the repair of a severed nerve (which resembles the cut end of a telephone cable only thousands of times smaller) or the reconstruction of a paper-thin ocular muscle.

In the realm of plastic surgery, the unthinkable is now possible. Before the advent of this awesome technology, the world was a different place. If a woman had had a radical mastectomy followed by irradiation, she bore her scars in silence. A patient with a resected jaw withdrew from society, and a patient with a severed hand received a prosthesis.

We now move large areas of healthy tissue—skin, muscle, and sometimes even bone—from one part of the body to virtually any other part of the body where it is needed. We can do this because, through use of the operating microscope, we are now able to connect the tiny, microscopic arteries, veins, and nerves of the donor tissue to their counterparts in the recipient area. This free transfer of tissue allows breasts to be reconstructed, jaws lost to cancer to be rebuilt, and severed hands to be attached.

Almost monthly, plastic surgery journals report on new applications utilizing microsurgical technology for the treatment of yet another "impossible" problem.

The big question about the future of plastic surgery is likely to be answered in a *small* way—through microsurgery.

Endoscopy

The endoscope consists of two basic parts: (1) a tubular probe, fitted with a tiny camera and a bright light, which is inserted through a small incision, and (2) a viewing screen, very much like a computer monitor or television screen, which magnifies the transmitted image.

Using this enhanced endoscopic image, the surgeon is able to maneuver surgical instruments—scalpel, scissors, and forceps—which are inserted through a second, separate incision.

This technology has been used by specialists in general surgery and orthopedics for decades. Only recently has endoscopy been applied to plastic surgery. As more and more applications are investigated and its merits evaluated, its use in this field will become clearer.

The major advantage to the endoscopic approach to surgery is that operations can be performed through very small incisions. This alone reduces risk of nerve damage. Additionally, because less tissue is disturbed, bruising, swelling, and bleeding are minimized. Not surprisingly, this makes recovery easier for the patient. The use of the endoscope is being evaluated in a variety of reconstructive procedures, including nasal sinus drainage operations, nasal sinus polyp removal, and carpal tunnel release.

Following are some cosmetic uses of endoscopy.

Abdominoplasty

The endoscopic approach is used in patients who only require tightening of muscles. This is not a recommended application in patients who have excess skin.

Breast Augmentation

Insertion of some breast implants through small incisions in the navel or axilla is another potential application. Also, this technique may be used to evaluate the condition of implants already in place and to correct capsular contracture.

Face-Lift

Endoscopy is being evaluated for minor correction of facial laxity. It does not replace the traditional face-lift but may prove to be of assistance in positioning facial implants.

Forehead-Lift

This is the most widely employed cosmetic application of the endoscopic technique to a plastic surgery procedure. Multiple small incisions in the hairline are used instead of the traditionally utilized ear-to-ear incision for correction of brow ptosis and forehead wrinkling. If this proves to be successful, the advantage to patients with thinning hair is substantial.

If you are interested in endoscopic plastic surgery, check with your local medical center for the names of plastic surgeons who are accredited to perform these procedures.

Laser Plastic Surgery

Overview

If the word *laser* conjures up images of a powerful magical beam used by an intergalactic warrior, you would be halfway on track.

Laser (light amplification by stimulated emission of radiation) is, indeed, a powerful beam, but it's certainly not magic. This device produces a beam of nonspreading, monochromatic, visible light. This beam concentrates high energy to a pinpoint area, vaporizing that area while leaving surrounding tissues undamaged.

There are many types of laser with a variety of applications. They are frequently categorized by the gas or crystal used to produce the beam. For example, there are carbon dioxide (CO_2), argon, copper vapor, and many others. Each has a specific application.

Laser holds great potential for plastic surgery; however, it must still be regarded as an emerging technology. In reconstructive plastic surgery, the argon and Q switched ruby laser have proven useful in treating port wine stains of the face as well as other vascular conditions. In cosmetic surgery, the carbon dioxide laser is often used in skin resurfacing. Depending upon the type and location, tattoo removal may require a combination of lasers. Another cosmetic surgery application is in the area of blepharoplasty.

Laser Resurfacing/Tattoo Removal

Also known as the laser peel, this technique employs the carbon dioxide or similar laser to vaporize, or ablate, the outer layers of damaged skin, or, in the case of tattoos, the layers containing pigment. Once these layers are removed, new cells form, providing a smoother, tighter skin surface.

The best candidates for this procedure are men and women of all ages, ideally with fair, nonoily skin. Dark-complected patients run the risk of pigmentation change, which may be permanent. Patients who are being treated with Accutane® or have used it recently are discouraged from trying laser resurfacing. Similarly, individuals prone to keloid scar formation are not good candidates.

Laser resurfacing poses the risks of burns from the heat of the laser itself, scarring, and changes in pigmentation. An individual who is prone to herpes infections (cold sores) may require antiviral medication because laser resurfacing can activate a herpes infection. Less frequent but serious problems from laser resurfacing include ectropion and corneal injury. Recovery time after laser resurfacing may last months to as long as a year for resolution of post-treatment redness. Some patients report that they experience sensitivity to sun, wind, and salt spray two years after resurfacing.

There is a significant learning curve for laser use. Check with your medical center for names of physicians amply qualified to perform laser procedures. Be aware of any hype or pressure to have a laser procedure. Laser equipment is very expensive for the doctor. Fees will vary.

The procedure itself is commonly performed under local anesthesia with sedation. The length of the procedure is directly proportional to the size of the area being treated. The treated area will then be covered with a protective ointment. Some surgeons apply a bandage, which is left on for five to ten days.

It may take as long as a week for your new skin to appear. During this time, you will have varying degrees of crusting, which will separate by day ten. At this point, you will be applying a protective ointment and should expect to be pink.

After about two weeks, you will be able to apply camouflage makeup. As mentioned, pinkness may persist for several months, and you will require conscientious sunblock protection.

Results and recovery vary with the depth of the laser treatment and should be compared with other resurfacing modalities, such as chemical peels. Treated areas are usually smoother and more evenly pigmented. This is usually a one-time procedure.

Laser Blepharoplasty

Laser is being used as an adjunct or sometimes as a substitute for the surgical scalpel in performing upper and lower blepharoplasty. Advocates of this technique feel that there is reduced postoperative bruising and swelling. Critics assert that there is no significant advantage over standard blepharoplasty and the added expense and risk involved with laser procedures is not justified. These risks include ectropion and corneal injury. Both sides agree that the long-term results are identical.

Ultrasound

Ultrasound technology harnesses energy waves, similar to sound waves but higher in frequency and not perceptible to the human ear. When this sonic energy is directed at tissue, it is converted to heat energy. At lower concentrations, this can be used diagnostically as in prenatal examination. At higher concentrations, the ultrasound energy disrupts cells, causing them to break down. A pioneering ultrasonic application was in breaking up kidney stones that previously required surgical removal.

The current application of this technology to plastic surgery is in the area of liposuction. Initially, by transmitting ultrasound through a wand connected to an aspirator, the plastic surgeon emulsifies fat by a process called cavitation. Cell membranes are disrupted, releasing triglycerides and free fatty acids in what appears as liquid fat. This liquid is aspirated, leaving other structures, such as blood vessels, unaltered.

Ultrasound assisted liposuction (UAL) is used when large areas need to be treated. It is not employed in treating areas such as the knees or under the chin as the incisions required are larger than those needed for conventional liposuction.

A skin protector is needed at the incision site to prevent a burn to that area. Hyperthermia, an abnormal elevation in body tissue temperature, can cause scarring and promote infection. In response to this, new instruments are being designed in an effort to make this process cooler.

Time required for UAL is longer than for standard liposuction. Also, the cost is considerably greater. (At this time, the necessary equipment costs the doctor approximately $45,000.) This procedure cannot be performed in patients with cardiac pacemakers as the ultrasound may interfere with the pacemaker function.

As with all new technologies, this, too, should be considered as under investigation. Again, there is a significant learning curve for the surgeon and the complications inherent in this procedure are potentially serious, the most dramatic being accidental skin perforation by the ultrasound wand.

The trend is toward development of hollow probes that allow the fat to be emulsified and aspirated simultaneously. Presently, this is a two-step process in which fat is emulsified and then aspirated.

The most recent advancement in ultrasound-assisted liposuction is the external application or transmission of sound waves. Preliminary reports on this application, which received FDA approval in early fall 1997, are very encouraging as it eliminates most of the problems with the internal-wand technique.

Glossary

~

Abdominoplasty See standard abdominoplasty and mini abdominoplasty.

Adipose tissue Fat.

Ala nasi The outer wing-shaped wall of the nostril.

Alar nasal cartilage The wing-shaped connective tissue that makes up the tip of the nose.

Alar rim The border of the nostril.

Alphahydroxy acids (AHAs) The mildest of the chemical peel formulas, alphahydroxy acids include glycolic, lactic, fruit acids, etc., and they are used to improve skin texture and reduce fine wrinkles as well as mild irregularities in pigmentation. They are of limited value in treatment of deep wrinkles, severely uneven pigmentation, and scars.

Anabolic steroids A family of drugs with properties known to build body tissues, most notably muscles. In high doses, these drugs are converted by the body into feminizing hormones, which accounts for breast development in males and a host of other side effects, including acne and liver damage.

Anesthesia Loss of sensation in the body induced by administration of a type of drug known as an *anesthetic*. Types of anesthesia generally used in plastic surgery procedures include: *local anesthesia* (the injection of an anesthetic to numb the area being treated), *local with sedation* (medication administered by vein to induce sleep, followed by an injection of an anesthetic to numb the area being treated), and *general anesthesia* (an anesthetic gas administered to induce sleep with a ventilator to assist breathing). In many operations, regardless of the chosen anesthetic, your doctor will also use a local anesthetic with epinephrine, a vascular constrictor, to reduce bleeding during the operation and aid in controlling postoperative pain.

Antihelix   The inner fold in the cartilage that gives the outer ear its shape.

Areola   The pigmented area around the nipple.

Augmentation mammoplasty   Breast augmentation using implants.

Axilla/axillae (pl.)   The armpit(s).

Bifid lobule   A torn earlobe.

Blepharoplasty   A cosmetic surgical procedure performed on the eyelids.

Breast implant   A silicone rubber shell filled with either silicone gel or inflated with a saline solution.

Canula   A small, hollow tube. In liposuction, it is inserted into the skin through one or more tiny incisions near the area to be suctioned. Attached to a syringe or vacuum pressure unit, the canula is guided by the surgeon to aspirate unwanted fat.

Capsule   Scar tissue that grows around implants or any foreign body. Any time a foreign substance is placed in the body, the body's response is to try to wall it off by forming a scar, or capsule, around that object.

Cartilage   The connective tissue (gristle) that forms the outer ear.

Cauliflower ears   An acquired deformity of the ear resulting from an undrained accumulation of blood usually caused by a blow to the ear; also known as boxer's ear.

Cellulite   A nonmedical term used to describe fatty deposits that give the skin an uneven, dimpled texture.

Chemical peel   A nonspecific term used to describe chemabrasion by any of a wide variety of agents that remove the superficial layer(s) of the skin in a controlled fashion. The result is a smoother, more evenly textured, and more evenly pigmented skin surface.

Cilia   Eyelashes.

Collagen   The major protein of connective tissue that makes up the foundation of skin and other tissues. When extracted from animal skin, it is used as an injectable filler to plump depressed areas or augment deficient areas of the skin. It is not administered to pregnant women, patients who are allergic to beef or bovine products, patients who suffer from autoimmune diseases, or those who are allergic to lidocaine, the local anesthetic mixed with the collagen.

Conjunctiva   The inner lining of the eyelids.

Conchal cartilage excess   A congenital condition in which there is too much cartilage in the lower portion of the ear, making the base of the ear stick out.

Cornea   The clear, sensitive covering of the pupil.

Corneal abrasion   A scratch of the cornea that causes intense pain and may result in visual impairment if not treated appropriately.

Corneal ulceration   A painful, crater-shaped interruption of the corneal surface caused by dry eye, which may lead to infection, scarring, and visual impairment if not treated appropriately.

Cosmetic plastic surgery   Also known as *aesthetic* or *esthetic* plastic surgery; includes operations performed to reshape normal structures in the body in order to improve appearance.

Craniofacial   A term relating to both soft tissues of the face and the underlying bony tissues of the skull.

Diastasis recti   The separation of the abdominal muscles, usually as a result of pregnancy or massive weight gain.

Dermabrasion   A technique of mechanical buffing of the skin, much like the sanding of a piece of wood, to remove the superficial layer(s) of the skin in a controlled fashion. This procedure is generally reserved for more serious skin problems and may be combined with a chemical peel or other plastic surgery procedures. The result is a smoother, more evenly textured, and more evenly pigmented skin surface.

Dermaplaning   A technique to remove superficial skin in layers using a dermatome, a mechanical device much like an electric razor. This is reserved for more serious skin problems.

Dermato lipectomy   Surgical removal of excess skin and fat.

Dog ear deformity   A mound of excess skin located at the extremes of an incision. Frequently self-limiting, if it persists, it may require a minor skin revision performed under local anesthesia three months after the initial operation.

Dry eye Inadequate lubrication of the eyeball due to exposure (lagophthalmos) or decreased tear production, which can lead to corneal ulceration.

Ectropion   A term used to describe the eversion or contraction of the lower eyelid resulting in scleral show; a condition also called bloodhound eyes.

Endoscope   A fiber-optic instrument that consists of two basic parts: (1) a tubular probe, fitted with a tiny camera and a bright light, which is inserted through a small incision, and

(2) a viewing screen, very much like a computer monitor or television screen, which magnifies the transmitted image.

Endoscopy   A fiber-optic technology that allows a surgeon to view images of the body's internal structures through very small incisions using a device called an *endoscope.*

Entropion   A term used to describe the inversion of the lower eyelid, which causes the lashes to rub against the eyeball.

Epinephrine   A neurohormone with many actions, used frequently in plastic surgery procedures for its ability to constrict small blood vessels and reduce intraoperative bleeding and prolong the effects of local anesthetics.

Excision   The act of cutting out. A surgical procedure to totally remove a tumor or scar.

Fat   Adipose tissue.

Fascia   Fibrous tissue that is found throughout the body beneath the skin. It encloses muscles and groups of muscles and separates and anchors several tissue layers of the body.

Flap operations   These procedures involve lifting a segment of tissue, keeping the bood and nerve supplies attached, and rotating it into an alternative position.

Gigantomastia   A medical term used to describe extremely large breasts.

Gortex   A lightweight, durable synthetic fiber used as a tissue filler.

Glabellar frown lines   The vertical creases between the eyebrows.

Graft   Living tissue moved from one part of the body to another. In the case of hair transplants, round-shaped *punch grafts* usually contain ten to fifteen hairs. A *minigraft* contains two to four hairs; a *micrograft,* one to two. *Slit grafts,* which are inserted into slits created in the scalp, contain four to ten grafts each. *Strip grafts*, which are long and thin, contain thirty to forty hairs.

Graves' disease   Hyperthyroidism.

Gynecomastia   Male breast enlargement.

Hydroquinone   A prescription bleaching agent, commonly used with Retin-A or AHA treatments for management of irregularities in skin pigmentation.

Hypertrophic scar   A medical term used to describe a widened or enlarged scar that remains within the boundaries of the initial injury or incision.

Hypospadias   A relatively common congenital anomaly in which the urethra does not extend to the end of the penis and opens elsewhere on the shaft.

Inframammary fold   The crease below the breast.

Injectable filler Any of several substances used to plump up a depressed area of the skin, such as a scar, or augment a deficient area.

Jowls   A term used to describe lax skin and pockets of fat that blunt the jawline.

Keloid   A hypertrophic scar that has outgrown the boundaries of the initial injury. This occurs when the body continues to manufacture collagen after a wound has healed. The keloid scar is often redder, thicker, and harder than surrounding skin. It is often annoyingly itchy.

Lagophthalmos   Inability to fully close the upper eyelid. It is transient in most cases because of postoperative swelling. A rare but more serious problem is lagophthalmos due to contracture, or shortening, of the upper eyelid muscles or skin. This condition may require surgical correction.

Laser   Light amplification by stimulated emission of radiation; a monochromatic, visible light that concentrates high energy to a pinpoint area, vaporizing that area while leaving surrounding tissues undamaged.

Laser assisted liposuction   An experimental technology using light energy to break up fat for removal.

Laser peel a.k.a. laser resurfacing   Use of laser to vaporize damaged skin while leaving surrounding tissues undamaged.

Lidocaine   Lidocaine hydrochloride; a common local anesthetic.

Limited liposuction   Also called spot or lunch hour liposuction. Small, specific fatty areas are treated, removing one to two cups of fat.

Liposuction a.k.a. standard liposuction   Liposuction treatment of a larger area, such as the abdomen or buttocks and thighs, removing one to two liters of fat.

Liquid silicone   In the early 1960s, injections of liquid silicone were used for breast augmentation. It was later disapproved for human use by the Food and Drug Administration (FDA) in 1965.

Lop ear deformity   A congenital condition in which the top of the ear flops forward, resulting from an unfurling of the antihelix. Also known as rabbit ears.

Mammography   Breast X ray. A diagnostic tool used not only to detect tumors but also to distinguish fat and glandular tissue.

Mammoplasty   Surgical procedure performed on the breast.

Marionette lines   A term used to describe vertical creases extending from the corners of the mouth to the jaw.

Mastectomy   Breast removal.

Mastopexy   Breast lift.

Milia   Skin cysts that look like whiteheads, which may form in a resurfaced area or along a suture line.

Mini abdominoplasty   This is the more commonly performed procedure to correct stretched muscles from the pubis to the *umbilicus,* with or without excess skin resection. It is frequently combined with liposuction.

Molded silicone   Semisolid silicone that is easily shaped for use as implants, especially for calves, chest, buttocks, and face.

Nasal dorsum   The ridge of the nose formed of bone at the bridge and cartilage at the tip.

Nasal septum   The wall dividing the nasal cavity into halves, formed posteriorly of bone and anteriorly of cartilage.

Nasolabial fold   The crease extending from the side of the nostril to the corner of the mouth.

Orbit   Eye socket.

Otoplasty   A medical term referring to the surgical correction of an ear deformity.

Palpebral fold   The crease in the upper eyelid.

Panniculectomy   A surgical procedure that removes large quantities of redundant skin and its underlying fat. Most often this operation is performed on the abdomen to remove the apron of fat and skin; however, the term refers to any area of the body, such as the arms.

Pannus   From the Latin meaning *piece of cloth.* Used to refer to any area of excess fat and skin, most commonly the apron of fat and skin hanging from the abdomen and the flabby, winglike underarm.

Pectoral muscles   The primary muscles of the chest.

Phenol   The strongest of the chemical solutions used to remove wrinkles in the skin.

Physiologic saline   This is a saltwater solution, the same as IV saline. Closely resembling the solution that makes up approximately 71 percent of the human body, it is used to inflate breast implant shells to desired size.

Platysmal bands   Cords of the platysma muscle that extend from the jaw to the collarbone on either side of the neck.

Ptosis   Drooping or sagging. Brow ptosis refers to the sagging of the eyebrow below the level of the upper rim of the eye socket. Weakness or detachment of the levator muscle, which raises the upper lid, usually is the cause of upper eyelid ptosis. When referring to breasts, it usually describes breasts after pregnancy.

Reconstructive plastic surgery   Surgical procedures performed on *abnormal* structures of the body. These abnormalities may be caused by congenital defects, such as cleft lip and palate, or trauma, burns, infections, tumors, or disease. Surgery improves function and, when possible, approximates normal appearance.

Resect/resection   To cut off or cut out.

Retin-A   A prescription medication derived from vitamin A, prescribed commonly by a dermatologist in the treatment of acne and used frequently as an exfoliating pretreatment for chemical peels. Its therapeutic effect beyond acne control is stimulation of skin growth, resulting in smoother, healthier-appearing skin.

Rhinoplasty   Reconstructive or plastic surgery of the nose.

Rhytid   A wrinkle.

Rhytidectomy   The surgical procedure to remove wrinkles; a face-lift.

Scalp expansion (skin expansion)   First stage of a two-stage procedure to bring hair together at the crown. A balloonlike tissue expander is inserted beneath the scalp and inflated in weekly treatments over several weeks to stretch and loosen skin.

Scalp reduction   Second stage of scalp reconstruction or hair restoration following scalp expansion and, on occasion, flap surgery. A segment of bald scalp is removed and skin is brought together and sutured to cover the bald area.

Scar   The connective tissue remnant of the body's healing process in response to injury.

Scar revision   A term used to describe a variety of procedures, including chemical peels, injections of steroids, or surgical revisions used to improve the appearance and/or orientation of scars.

Sclera   The white part of the eyeball.

Scleral hematoma   A black-and-blue mark on the sclera that appears as a cherry red spot that resolves over a two- to three-week period.

Scleral show   A result of ectropion, caused by the retraction of the lower eyelid, which exposes the sclera below the pupil of the eye when looking straight ahead.

Sclerotherapy   A technique for treating spider veins, telangiectasias, or sunburst varicosities by injecting a solution that collapses the vessel.

Septoplasty   Reconstructive surgery of the nasal septum.

Silicone gel   This is a jellylike silicone rubber used in early breast implants. Silicone gel–filled implants are available only through controlled FDA studies and in special cases of reconstruction.

Skin expansion   See scalp expansion.

SMAS (submusculo aponeurotic segment) face-lift   A two-tiered face-lift procedure, the major component of which is tightening of the connective tissue and muscular layer of the face before redraping the skin.

Spider veins   Nonessential dilated veins that lie just under the skin.

Standard abdominoplasty   A surgical procedure that removes excess fat and skin from the abdomen. Frequently, this includes tightening severely stretched abdominal muscles, from the pubis to the breastbone, and repositioning the *umbilicus* (belly button). This requires a transverse incision, usually extending from hip to hip, and an umbilical incision to reposition the navel.

Subciliary Incision   An incision placed on the outside of the lower eyelid, just below the eyelashes, for removal of excess skin and fat.

Submental fat   The fat found under the chin, commonly associated with double chins.

Sunburst varicosities   Tiny, nonessential veins that lie close to the skin in a pattern resembling sunbursts; spider veins.

Telangiectasias   Tiny, nonessential veins that lie close to the skin without a specific pattern; spider veins.

Tragus   A tonguelike projection of cartilage in front of the opening of the ear canal.

Transconjunctival incision   An incision placed on the inside of the lower eyelid for removal of fat.

Trichloroacetic acid (TCA)   Most commonly used for medium-depth peeling, TCA is commonly used to treat fine surface wrinkles, uneven pigmentation, and superficial blemishes.

Tumescent/tumescence   A liposuction technique that introduces large amounts of dilute anesthetic solution into the area to be treated. The fluid causes the area to balloon, ensuring minimal discomfort to the patient, making aspiration of the fat easier, and reducing postoperative discomfort.

Ultrasound   A developing technology that utilizes sound waves to break up the fat for easier removal in ultrasound assisted liposuction (UAL).

Umbilicus   Navel.

W-plasty; Z-plasty   Common surgical techniques used to lengthen contracted scar tissue and reorient scars so that they more closely conform to natural skin lines and creases, making them less noticeable. The letters describe the incision pattern.

Resources

~

The Plastic Surgery Information Service, sponsored by the American Society of Plastic and Reconstructive Surgeons and the Plastic Surgery Education Foundation, offers a Web site to provide information on various aspects of cosmetic and reconstructive plastic surgery. The Plastic Surgery Information Service Web address is http://www.plastic-surgery.org.

Topics include:

❖ Overview/tips for using the Web site

❖ Finding a plastic surgeon

❖ Frequently asked questions about plastic surgery

❖ The surgery (information about plastic surgery procedures)

❖ In the news (a look at plastic surgeons in the news)

❖ The media center (a reference library for media)

❖ Professional information

❖ Links (where to find additional resources)

❖ Feedback (tell the service what you think about the Web site and plastic surgery)

❖ What's new (recent additions to the Web site)

❖ American Society of Plastic and Reconstructive
    Surgeons, Inc.
  444 E. Algonquin Road
  Arlington Heights, IL 60005-4664
  Telephone: 847-228-9900; 1-800-635-0635

❖ American Board of Plastic Surgeons, Inc.
  7 Penn Center, Suite 400
  1635 Market St.
  Philadelphia, PA 19103
  Telephone: 215-587-9322

❖ American Academy of Facial Plastic and Reconstructive
    Surgery
  1101 Vermont Ave. NW, Suite 404, Dept. MC
  Washington, DC 20005
  Telephone: 1-800-332-3223

❖ American Medical Association
  515 N. State St.
  Chicago, IL 60610
  Telephone: 312-464-5000

❖ American Society for Aesthetic Plastic Surgery, Inc.
  444 E. Algonquin Road
  Arlington Heights, IL 60005
  Telephone: 847-228-9274

Also contact your local medical society, hospitals, and medical centers.

Index

~

Page numbers in *italics* refer to figures in the text.

About the Author

~

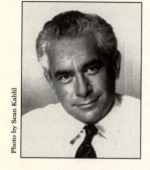

Photo by Sean Kahlil

RICHARD A. MARFUGGI, M.D., F.A.C.S., is a board-certified plastic surgeon who has been practicing plastic and reconstructive surgery in New York City since 1983. He is a member of the American Society of Plastic and Reconstructive Surgeons (ASPRS) and is a fellow of the American College of Surgeons (FACS).

An honor graduate of The College of the Holy Cross in Worcester, Massachusetts, he received his medical degree from the University of Vermont College of Medicine and completed his general surgery training at the University Health Center Hospitals in Pittsburgh and the Eastern Virginia Graduate School of Medicine in Norfolk.

Dr. Marfuggi completed his specialty training in plastic and reconstructive surgery at the Institute for Reconstructive Plastic Surgery at the New York University Medical Center, where he was among the last residents selected by the famed pioneer in the field, Dr. John Marquis Converse.

Prior to conducting research in wound healing at The Yale New Haven Medical Center, Dr. Marfuggi studied pediatric cardiothoracic surgery at The Hospital for Sick Children, Great Ormond Street, in London, England.

Dr. Marfuggi's professional affiliations include the American Society of Plastic and Reconstructive Surgeons, the American College of Surgeons, the New York State Medical Society, the Harbison Surgical Society, the John Marquis Converse Plastic Surgery Society, and the C. F. Reynolds

Medical Historical Society. He has served on national committees for the American Society of Plastic and Reconstructive Surgeons and has lectured widely. He has been honored for his scientific presentations and publications by such prestigious groups as the American College of Surgeons and the American Society of Plastic and Reconstructive Surgeons.

With offices in Manhattan and in Denville, New Jersey, where he is codirector of the Institute for Plastic Surgery, he has staff privileges at New York's Center for Specialty Care and the Cabrini Medical Center and New Jersey's Morristown Memorial Hospital, Elizabeth General Medical Center, and Northwest Covenant Medical Center.

Dr. Marfuggi has been a consultant on network television and radio and has appeared on numerous local and national talk radio and television programs. He has been featured in *The New York Times* and other national newspapers and in such magazines as *Ladies' Home Journal, Allure, Vogue, Marie Claire, Mirabella, Cosmopolitan, W, Men's Health,* and *Genre.*